Infinity Health Manual

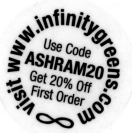

Infinity Health Manual

The Essentials for Longevity, Weight Loss, & the Mind...Simplified

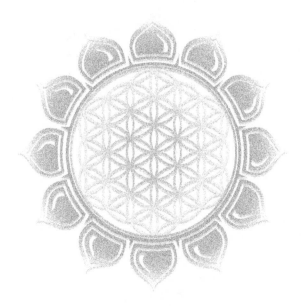

Billy Merritt

Infinity Health Manual
The Essentials for Longevity,
Weight Loss, & the Mind...Simplified

Billy Merritt

FIRST EDITION

ISBN: 978-0-692-88775-2 (print)
ISBN: 978-0-692-88776-9 (ebook)

Library of Congress Control Number: 2017907349

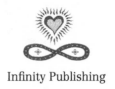

Infinity Publishing

Contents

Acknowledgements

This book has happened thanks to a number of people for whom I am so very grateful. First, I want to say thank you to The Ashram—the entire staff and especially Cat. Thank you for allowing me to utilize my nutritive principles in the design of The Ashram's dietary protocols. Also, a thank you to the guests, who were all such wonderful people, always asking great questions in my classes which inspired me to research the secrets of natural health deeper and deeper. Watching people enhance their lives by living this information is why this is my passion. And a big thank you to Jerry Payne, my editor, who did such awesome work! This book would not be anything near what it is without him. My parents and siblings, too. Their moral support and feedback were essential. With their encouragement, they were the ones who helped inspire me to walk this path in the first place. And lastly, thank you to Arbear my golden retriever who was right by my side for the entire journey of writing this book! The best pup ever!

PS. This book is dedicated to YOU. I have seen this content change the lives of thousands of people and I am honored to have you on the journey. So here we go!

Introduction

Dear Friend,

The potential wellbeing that is at our fingertips is no less than extraordinary. Under the shadow of the modern, less-than-healthy lifestyles, however, it's simply been forgotten. But how to live a genuinely healthy way of life is part of our intuitive wisdom. It's an intelligence in our genes honed from the many thousands of years that we have evolved whilst nourishing body, mind, and spirit with the unquestionably powerful elements of pure food, fresh air, water, and sunshine. Living a healthy life creates a quality of experience for which no one has ever regretted spending the time and effort. The wellbeing of mind and body is invaluable. And the value, as great as it already is, can yet become even greater as we walk this path. In this book, I have mapped out what I've experienced to be the essential lifestyle protocols for manifesting our greatest self-hood. This is a quest of making the mind and body superhuman. The potential is truly awesome, yet little-known. I can guarantee you that living the information within this book will be reflected by enhancing your longevity, energy, ability to heal, clarity of thought and *even* your happiness. And weight loss, too, if that's something you wish for!

The reality is we live in an age with increased rates of obesity, diabetes, heart disease, cancer, and a plethora of autoimmune diseases. Nothing in this book is meant to be a silver bullet for ailments, but I firmly believe that the principles herein can collectively lead to a lifestyle where the threat and discomfort of these diseases can at least be substantially reduced. And in many instances, complete healing may be possible. This is also a topic we'll discuss. The body's healing abilities, when properly supported, are nothing less than awesome.

The reason that what is possible with our health has become underestimated in the modern world is because many people don't have anything to compare their lifestyles to. Most people of the Western world have been living in the status quo all their lives. And the reality is the modern "status quo lifestyle" is weak, relative to what is possible. We've neglected the diet and lifestyle that make us truly strong and healthy. Further, we have not adapted to the pollutants of the modern way of life (and never will) like processed foods, environmental toxins, household pollutants, and chemical additives in food and water. Not to mention stress. Physical, emotional, and mental stress put a collective strain on the organs and the nervous system, making the body and mind weaker. Aging is not as much a matter of time as it is the rate at which the body and mind are allowed to atrophy. The concept of living the anti-aging lifestyle is truly legitimate. Each healthy thing we do for ourselves perpetuates us more and more in the right direction and is reflected as a stronger selfhood. We're talking potential results of physical *and* mental well-being! A truly healthy body supports a healthy neurological system and thus a healthy mind (which then takes better care of the body). The scale of what's possible is awesome.

How did I come across this awareness of what the body is capable of? It was no accident. Much of it began with my journey of searching to heal myself from a rare condition of bleeding vessels in my brain that was causing seizures every day. During this time I devoted my life to discovering ways the body can become empowered to heal itself.

But even before my own healing journey I had an understanding of the intimate connection between health and lifestyle. It wasn't completely new territory for me. Until I began having the seizures, I'd been working at the Ashram Health Retreat in the Santa Monica Mountains of Southern California. The Ashram is known for enhancing people's physical and mental well-being by providing a nutrition and exercise program of awesome precision. It's a week-long program that every day includes a hike of at least ten miles (a total of seventy miles for the week), two fitness classes, a pool class, and two yoga classes—all of which I believe to be made possible by the truly wonderful diet. Highly acclaimed and world-famous, the Ashram has catered to the likes of Oprah Winfrey, Cindy Crawford, Colin Farrell, Catherine Zeta Jones, and a host of other people, including regular folks just like you and me, all looking to make a real difference in their lives.

For eight years, I taught nutrition at the Ashram, teaching the protocols used in the program. I also devised the diet. The diet was (and still is) a big part of what enabled the guests to engage in the rigorous activities of the Ashram. People were able to do things that beforehand would have seemed impossible and, for many, probably were.

Let it be known, however, that I wasn't always so knowledgeable about nutrition and healthy living. As a kid, I ate more than a fair amount of junk food. Thankfully my parents at least made me eat my fruits and vegetables. But even healthy foods don't negate the wear and tear from high consumption of candy bars and Kool-Aid. When I got to college, I upped my intake of other common junk foods including the classics like fried foods, pizza, and hamburgers, along with a steady diet of French fries, ice cream, and baked sweets. And I wondered why I didn't always feel so hot. I even got a little chubby around the waist. In my mind the dots between diet and health just didn't connect.

It was after college, when I started preparing my own food, that it began to click in my mind the connection between what I was eating and my sense of health. I started catching on to the benefits of eating well, very simply because of a renewed sense of vitality that came with a better diet. In my early twenties I began a career as a professional climbing guide, and I know I could not have performed the physical labor that was involved without a genuinely healthy diet. Then, during a climbing trip to Nepal and Thailand, I spent part of my time at a health retreat where I really *lived* a comprehensive healthy lifestyle, to a much greater degree than I ever had before. How I felt while living this life was like flipping a switch, and I knew I'd never look at life the same way again, nor would I go back to the ways of a not-so-healthy diet.

So by the time of my brain diagnosis a healthy way of life had already become a passion. During this time I had also introduced healing arts into my life, too, some of which I will share with you later in the book. It was with my comprehensive healing lifestyle that little by little, my health came back. This represented clear proof to me that, with the proper support, the body is better at healing itself than we give it credit for. It's pretty awesome, our potential. Really my condition has been an extraordinary blessing in disguise. I call it a terrible privilege. I've learned that even if the condition is a genetic one, like mine, lifestyle can trump genes when given the chance. But the fact that we *all* have the potential for truly enhancing our health remains largely unknown, especially in the Western world. I had the opportunity to witness it firsthand with those who would come to the Ashram and leave as different people. It was always an awakening experience and nothing less than jaw dropping—for them *and* me.

Why do I mention all of this? Because I want to let you know that the information I have to share with you comes from experience—experience that has made the material in this book my driving passion. It's my very life. I'd like to make this material a part of your life, too.

In these pages you'll find practical knowledge that can help you regardless of your body type and present condition. These are dietary and lifestyle adjustments that can be effective for anyone. And I'll help you find a way to take the principles herein and integrate them into your life. You'll discover what I discovered on my life-healing journey: if you give your body the elite nutritive and lifestyle support, you'll uncover a healthier you. Most importantly, you'll feel the vitality and life-force that come with it.

But wait! This is about more than just physical health. It's mental health, too. Our diets and lifestyle affect us holistically. Nutrients support the body's organs and functions, which ultimately take care of the neurological system which, in turn, then better regulates the body. It's a cycle that produces mental well-being as well as physical well-being. Expect for this to be reflected in your mood, memory, and ability to think. Do you need any other reasons?

Hey, does all of this mean you can't have a slice of birthday cake if you're out with friends? Of course not. That's not what this book is about. We're talking about your overall lifestyle, not the occasional moment of socialization. Nobody wants to be the wet blanket at the party. But I will say this: when your friends and family pick up on your renewed life-force, generated by the principles you'll find in this book, they're going to find it very appealing. Radiant health is attractive. And you'll be leading by example without even trying. Without even saying a word, you can be a positive influence towards those around you.

So let's dig in. The good news is that this stuff is pretty easy to do. One could write volumes on health, but I've distilled the information here to what I've experienced to be the most effective protocols for the amount of effort they require. These are the tools that I watched revamp and enhance the health and vitality of everyone who went through the Ashram. I could even see the change in their skin and eyes. And the difference they would feel by the end of the week was always dramatic. I very much anticipate this information will do the same for you. And I think you'll find all of this a lot of fun, too. You might start out needing a little discipline to incorporate these principles, but I'm confident the rewards will be so apparent that the discipline will fast become desire. And, really, none of this is hard.

At the Ashram, I had the opportunity to watch thousands of people live these principles, and I've lived them myself. The question is, what would happen if *you* lived them? The sheer potential is intriguing, isn't it? Let's raise a few bars and see what happens!

Yours truly, and at your service always,

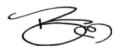

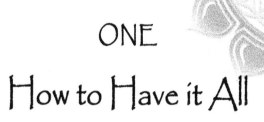

ONE

How to Have it All

Is it possible to have it all? A fit body, radiant skin, a strong immune system, a healthy mind, and *even* a satisfied palate?

The short answer? A definite "YES!"

There are a lot of principles in this book you'll learn to employ but let's start with the most basic: a fundamental key to your life-force and longevity is to add genuinely healthy foods to your diet. This, along with more fresh air, sunshine, and pure water, which we'll also discuss in this book.

The Big Picture

As for healthy foods, what are we talking about? Well, they're foods that are, for the most part, in an unprocessed, unrefined state—plus a few vitally important ones that should be part of *everyone's* diet. Today, adequate consumption of these foods has fallen *way* short in the average diet. Instead, a large percentage of the modern diet consists of processed foods (even foods that we may not think of as processed) such as breads, pastas, cereals, crackers, chips, other snack foods, and bottled drinks. These foods give the body very little of what it really needs.

And what does the body need? Nutrients! Vitamins, minerals, and enzymes from whole unprocessed foods! The old saying,

"You are what you eat," is more true than we might realize. New cells, the very substance we are made of, are being created every moment. Although it's largely imperceptible to the outside senses, our bodies are constantly changing, for good or for bad, based on what we're feeding ourselves. Every seven years, your body has all new cells. Except for the neurons in the brain, every cell gets replaced. That's the importance of rebuilding your body with the right stuff all the time. While so much of our population manages to get by on processed foods, seeming to defy the laws of nature, processed foods *do* have costs that most people are not aware of.

Overeat...Diet...Repeat

Without enough nutrient-dense foods the body fails to get what it needs: *vital nutritive life-support*. And because of this, the appetite remains unsatisfied. So then what do we do? We eat more. And it's more of the same processed stuff. It's a common flaw in the Western world. We overeat in an attempt to satisfy our appetites, and we overeat the wrong things. By nature, the body doesn't like to overeat for many reasons, of course the unfortunate outcome of obesity being an obvious one. And obesity isn't necessarily the worst of the potential outcomes either.

What's a typical response? To eat less. We diet. Most dieting is based on restraining the overall intake of calories to a specific amount based on body weight and number of pounds needing to be lost. This approach fails because it basically restrains a diet that is already nutrient deficient. The primary goal of weight loss may be achieved, but often at the expense of overall health, even at the cost of simply feeling good.

By the way, don't be bamboozled by the "low-fat" diets for weight loss. We'll talk more about fats in the next chapter. For now, here's a crucial reality check: when the low-fat diets began twenty years ago, Americans started to get fatter!

And dieting can only ever be a temporary solution at best because the body's metabolism slows down to compensate for the reduced fuel available. When the regular diet returns, the weight comes back due to the slowed metabolic rate—and sometimes with a vengeance. Processed foods really just make life harder. These foods have only recently become "familiar" and our bodies are confused about how much to eat. So we spend our time counting our calories and percentages of fat, protein, and carbohydrates. With the unprocessed foods, Mother Nature has all that taken care of for us.

Our bodies are incredibly intelligent and, by nature, aspire toward operating at a level of optimal strength and well-being. When we incorporate nutrient-dense foods in our diet, thereby getting what we really need, our bodies know it. Conversely our taste buds know to stay away from things in nature that could otherwise be toxic to our bodies. Unfortunately, in our modern day and age, the common foods are more about entertainment than nutrition. They're unfamiliar to our otherwise intelligent taste buds and beyond the scope of the body's instinctive wisdom. The modern diet is diverting us from what is genuinely healthy, and a hypnotic spell comes with it, making the body unaware it's headed down the wrong path. But it doesn't have to be that way; with the right understanding we can get back on course by listening to the intelligence of our bodies and re-training our taste buds.

So the win-win solution to any diet, whether the goal is weight loss, increased energy, or healing, is to add natural, unprocessed, nutrient-dense foods to your diet. It will unquestionably be reflected in numerous ways that will prove to be significant. And as your body's natural instincts will become revamped you'll by nature gravitate toward more of the genuinely healthy foods over time, and faster than you might think.

Multivitamins, Fortified Foods, Supplements, and Superfoods

What if you don't have time to prepare your own food? Or what if you just don't have a taste and liking for most vegetables? Well,

3

there's always multivitamins, right? Not necessarily. The human body has evolved over many thousands of years, nourished all along with nutrients from real foods. Only in recent years have we seen a departure from this vital relationship. There have been countless attempts at devising substitutes for nutrition from foods— multivitamins, nutrient isolates, and similar supplements. These are synthetically processed nutrients, and are for the most part, unfamiliar to the body, therefore offering little to no benefit. Some multivitamins advertise that they're made with plant foods but they still include nutrients synthetically created in labs! And what do I mean by "nutrients synthetically created"? These are derivatives from coal tar mixed with different varieties of genetically modified corn and hydrochloric acid. Huh? Who would really want to ingest *that*? Not me. Do a search on the web, and you will find very little information about this very topic. I have a hunch why.

Promoted as healthy, these "100% of your vitamins" products can, ironically, create a toxic load on the body, especially the kidneys. Multivitamins and other lab-formulated nutrients are no match for the *real* nutrients from foods, and, used long-term, could produce more harm than benefit. Note: even the most nutrient-rich plant-food diet won't give the body 100 percent of every vitamin and mineral the body needs in a day. Nor is it necessary. Many nutrients are fat soluble and are stored in the body, some even for years, like vitamin B-12 for example. Getting our nutrients from food is something the body has already perfected – not so, from artificial nutrients.

And let's not be fooled by thinking we're getting nutrients in the so-called fortified foods at the local supermarket. These are often the foods made with wheat flour that's "fortified" with thiamine, riboflavin, niacin, and iron. Why? Because these are the nutrients in the original wheat bran that are lost during the processing of wheat into a pulverized powder (a.k.a. flour). And because these nutrients are removed, food manufacturers put the lab-formulated versions back in. The end result is nothing healthy. Worse, this wheat flour, as we'll discuss later on, is in *many* foods—even those presented as "natural."

What about supplements? It's a broad subject with a whole world of different products, some of which can be great and some of which are terrible. Overusing supplements is a common theme. And with many, tolerance can easily build negating any value. The main idea with any supplements you're taking is to read the list of ingredients to be sure it's exclusively plant foods that are known to be genuinely healthy.

Superfoods

As you probably already know, there's a wide array of products that are referred to as superfoods. Superfoods qualify as a plant food that has some sort of a substantial nutritive element to it. Some of the common superfoods include chard, collard greens, parsley, broccoli, ginger, turmeric, pomegranate, and blueberries. Other superfoods, maybe lesser-known, include maca root, blue-green algae, goji berries, herbs like nettles or passion flower, and super-high antioxidant fruits like mangosteen, acerola cherry, and amla berry.

A significant advantage of superfoods is many haven't been subject to nutrient loss from the soil depletion that has resulted from modern, mass-agricultural methods. It's a tough reality check to consider that many fruits and vegetables don't have quite the same nutritive content they used to. This is part of where super-foods can play an important role. It's the lesser known superfoods harvested in their native environment that generally maintain their original nutrient-richness.

You may already know I'm a huge believer in superfoods. I mention this not to endorse my Infinity products specifically, but to let you know how important a diet of truly healthy foods is to me. I've made it my life's work. I've witnessed superfoods, after a decade of formulating them for the Ashram, demonstrate clearly their tremendous health-enhancing value. Of course there are literally thousands of medicinal herbs and superfoods; my point is to introduce you to the idea of bringing them into your life.

It should be noted here that, in the case you are working on healing a malady it's important to research your superfoods before taking them. Some may have just the effects you're looking for, while others could have the opposite. There are some superfoods that are blood thinners, for example, while there are others that are blood coagulators—the very *opposite*. Do your research to find the superfoods that are a fit for your state of health and what it is you're shooting for. Wikipedia (not product websites) can be an awesome resource for this purpose. Try a superfood on a trial and error basis to evaluate if you're noticing any effects. Are you getting the results you're looking for? Superfoods that are just right for you could offer significant benefit. Just their potential energizing effect alone can make superfoods a superior alternative to....

Caffeine

In my classes I would often get asked about caffeine. A rule of thumb is about one-hundred milligrams of caffeine is within the boundaries of healthy intake. That's a regular cup of coffee. For comparison, a serving of black tea is about fifty milligrams. Green tea has about half that much, which is still enough caffeine to be stimulating. The red flag in the world of caffeinated beverages is energy drinks! Stay away from them. These drinks can have upwards of two-hundred milligrams or more of caffeine. Yikes!

The truth is, there's no added stimulation much past a hundred milligrams. Maybe only some anxiety. The advantage for the energy drink companies is that this much caffeine becomes chemically addicting. No doubt that's at least part of their idea. And the FDA isn't helping. Unbelievably, the FDA advises that 200 milligrams is safe even for children! Don't allow yourself or your kids to go down that road. The thing to keep in mind with caffeine is it can be over-stimulating and even exhausting for the adrenals, and can actually rob you of energy in the long run. In most cases, *moderate* amounts of caffeine probably won't hurt. Personally, I have found that I definitely have more energy when I am caffeine-free. Still, I may have a cup of tea from time to time when I feel like I really need it. If you're a daily caffeine drinker, why not take a break to see how it goes? At first, you may feel draggy because the adrenals are recharging, but give it a few days and you'll likely feel the energy advantage.

GMO

Over the last thirty years our foods have been altered significantly. How? Foreign genes from other plants and animals have been inserted into the genes of the original plant food. DNA profiles have been restructured for the purpose of making foods grow faster and bigger, and more resistant to drought and bruising, as well as increasing the food's shelf life. GMO (Genetically Modified Organisms) now comprise the vast majority of our food supply.

Unfortunately the negatives of GMO foods outweigh the positives. The end result of a genetically modified food is simply this: it's a radically different product. For the most part, the calories and nutritive profiles of the genetically altered food are similar to the original, but there's a lot more to a food than just calories and nutrients. Genetic structures of food play a big role for a number of reasons.

It should be noted here that genetic engineering is somewhat mid-experiment. Whether genetic modification is linked to the plethora of modern health issues is simply unknown at this point, and not knowing the *long-term* effects on our health (and the environment) is deserving of serious attention. Genetic modification of foods is currently outlawed in thirty eight countries, all of which I trust to have plenty of intelligent people. Like them, I prefer to not put myself at risk in this GMO experiment, and my intuition tells me that maintaining a diet of primarily organic foods is well worth the extra cost. For me, there are particular foods where I can always tell the difference in the taste and texture between genetically modified and organic, and organic is always better.

Furthermore, most genetically engineered foods are grown with the use of pesticides. The job of pesticides of course is to kill things. GMO foods generally need pesticides because the plant's natural ability to defend itself from insects has been compromised by the residual holes left behind from its change in genetic structure. Ingesting even residual amounts of pesticides on a lifestyle basis is worthy reason for concern. Naturally, taking in pesticides doesn't lend itself well to our overall health. I strongly suggest going for foods that are *certified organic*. This means foods that have had no genetic modifications and that have not been treated with pesticides. For animal foods, it means that even the feed has been exclusively organic. As for the newly classified, "Non-GMO Verified" foods, while it's true they haven't been genetically modified, they can still contain pesticides. When will the day come when GMO foods or foods sprayed with pesticides have to be labeled as such? I think it would make a huge difference to the consumer if he or she was aware, when buying a food product, that "this product has been genetically modified and sprayed with chemicals."

In addition to seeking organic foods, always read the ingredients of the packaged products you're buying. There are a lot of processed foods out there that are billed as organic. Organic crackers, chips, cereals, breads, etc. Yes, they may be made from organic food, but they're still processed and therefore lacking the healthy nutritional value we're looking for. Unfortunately, the term "organic" has become weakened from many processed foods being labeled as such.

Along those lines, don't be fooled by the term "all natural." All this means is that the food product isn't artificially flavored or colored. But it can be genetically modified or treated with pesticides. For crying out loud, even high-fructose corn syrup is classified as "all natural"!

Salt

One more basic dietary topic I get asked a lot about is salt. Salt is among the important reasons to read ingredient labels. Listed on a product label as "salt," "table salt," or "iodized salt," it's salt that has likely been mined from the ground. Lesser-processed sea salt is a better option because sea salt has trace minerals which are lacking in the regular salt products. The problem with mined salt is it's exclusively sodium chloride with no minerals, and too much sodium chloride by itself can be de-mineralizing for the body. It's also been linked to high blood pressure and high water retention that only slow down the body's processes. Some sodium in our diet is essential for the conduction of electrical impulses that keep everything in the body ticking, but sodium is already in many plant foods, like celery for example. You don't need the common salt that's found in typical snack foods, sauces, flavors, dips, dressings, and similarly processed foods. Almost all of these packaged foods have salt added due to lack of flavor and for extending their shelf life. Take the processed salt products out of your diet. This, of course, means less processed and packaged foods in general. Read those labels and shop for products that use exclusively sea salt.

If and when adding salt to your food, Celtic sea salt is my first choice. It's the least processed of salt products, still has its original trace minerals, and is okay when used in small amounts. Himalayan salt is a fine option, too. Still, these natural salts can be overused. Just a pinch will do. Rather than too much salt in your food, up the flavor with herbs and spices.

Easier Than You Think

Your diet is a powerful avenue for quality of life enhancement. And honing its improvement is an ongoing life journey. As such, it's a matter of starting where you are and adding a few of the truly healthy foods to your daily routine. Don't overwhelm yourself with the idea of a complete diet overhaul. For many the body can reject this kind of radical change. Your tastes will gradually change in the favor of genuinely healthy foods, and your choices will gravitate in that direction. Remember that your intelligent taste buds will conspire on your behalf when you give them a chance with the right foods. And hopefully you'll find that this book will offer a steady progression of supportive information that'll help your shift toward a healthier life feel quite natural.

If this is new territory for you, then congratulations! Let's start simple. I have the perfect suggestions that I'll be sharing with you as we go, and you can find a whole section of recipes in the back. The point is, it's a lot easier to raise the quality of your diet than you might think. And you may just find the reward to be much greater than expected. I sure did.

Ready to learn more? In the next few chapters I'm going to disabuse you of what you thought you knew about fats, sugars, starches, and proteins. From there, we'll move on to other important subjects that might also challenge conventional wisdom. The thing to ponder here is what will life be like when we truly embrace a healthy diet and lifestyle? There is a pricelessness to the well-being we were destined to live, and I say we go for it.

TWO

The Skinny on Fats

I hope you're sitting down because I've got some news for you that might just be shocking. Ready? Eating fat does not necessarily make you fat. Furthermore, dropping fat from your diet doesn't necessarily make you lose weight. In fact, it can even have the opposite effect!

Ever wonder why, as a nation, we're getting fatter and fatter, and yet so many of us seem to be on "low-fat" diets? Something doesn't add up. Well, as most people know, there are healthy fats and unhealthy fats. But since "fat" is too often regarded as a cause of our obesity problem, we don't differentiate between the two the way we should. All fat is inherently seen as bad by many of us. But fat is essential to health. Like carbohydrates, it's fuel! And many vitamins and minerals are fat soluble which means that fat is required as the catalyst to break these nutrients down for the body to absorb. If you're on a low-fat diet for even just a couple weeks, you're likely to feel some negative effects. You can eat all the right nutrients, but if you don't have the right amount of fat to act as the catalyst to absorb the nutrients, you can actually become deficient in them.

Fats are also needed for healthy joints and connective tissues. And here's another plus: fats satisfy an appetite quickly to help prevent overeating. Ever sit down with a bag of low-fat chips and, before you know it, you've polished off the whole bag? You keep eating them because the body never feels satisfied. It's the same with all "low-fat" foods like crackers, bread, cereal, pasta, and other starchy foods. It's easy to overeat them. And then what does your body do with the overflow of the starchy calories? It stores them as...*fat!* One-hundred calories of the healthy fats (what you might find in an avocado, for instance), tends to be more satisfying to the body than one-hundred calories of carbohydrates, like found in grains. Same amount of calories, much different level of satiation.

Finally, did you know that the human brain is eighty percent fat? Not only have we become a nation of people getting fatter with our low-fat diets, we're potentially compromising our neurological health.

Unhealthy Fats

The answer is not to remove fat from your diet. The answer is to eat more *healthy* fats while avoiding the *unhealthy* ones. It's the unhealthy fats that are responsible, to a large degree, for obesity and its attendant diseases. Heart disease and diabetes are on the rise and unhealthy fat is a big culprit.

Unhealthy fats are everywhere. A little history lesson: back in the 1980s, food manufacturers came out with cheap ways to cook things. Suddenly we were all eating foods cooked in inexpensive oils like corn, canola, or safflower oil. These are expeller-pressed oils that become rancid even before you buy them, and they are guaranteed to make the thyroid, which governs your metabolism, weaker. These oils are what you find in common snack foods, bread, cereal, and similar processed foods.

Even worse is hydrogenated vegetable oil. Hydrogenated vegetable oil is produced by heating vegetable oil to 700 degrees and then filtering hydrogen gas through it. The oil becomes unstable at such high temperatures, thus allowing the hydrogen atoms to bond with the oil. The oil then cools to become a solid at room temperature, like butter. The process has a dangerous side effect: free radicals. What are free radicals? These are unstable molecules that roam around the body chipping particles from cell walls, which then create more free radicals. As you may know, eliminating free radicals is a vital role of antioxidants, found primarily in raw fruits and vegetables, which we'll talk about later.

Free radicals are produced from many sources other than unhealthy foods, including overexposure to sunlight, environmental toxicity, and even stress. So we ingest free radicals all the time. For the most part, it's okay because, as mentioned above, our bodies are designed to deal with them via antioxidants in our diet, fresh air, pure water, and rest. But most people consume too many unhealthy fats that contain these free radicals. And an excess amount of them can be costly to one's health in several ways. The deteriorating nature of free radicals is among the primary causes of aging. And they can also be a cause of mutated cell growth and a weakened immune system making the body vulnerable to cancer. Plus, free radicals almost always suppress the body's thyroid function and that, right there, is a big cause of obesity. You zap your thyroid and you zap your metabolism. Slow metabolism = weight gain.

To offset this, once oils like hydrogenated vegetable oil hit the market, we started reducing our intake of *all* fats. We started looking for low-fat alternatives and starving ourselves of the needed healthy fats and buying into the calorie-counting protocol as a discipline. That's a recipe tailor-made for failure.

The Right Fats

Fats come in two categories: saturated and unsaturated and it's easy to tell the difference. Saturated fat is solid at room temperature, unsaturated is liquid at room temperature. You need both. Yes, contrary to what you might have heard, you need even the saturated kind, as we'll discuss.

Unsaturated fats can be found in avocados, raw nuts and seeds, and oils that are liquid at room temperature, like olive oil. All processed oils should be cold-pressed. Cold-pressing means what the name implies: the oil is extracted under cool temperatures, thus protecting the potential health-creating qualities of the oil. But these are oils you don't want to cook with. Unsaturated fats break down when cooked. (This is why fried foods aren't good for us even if they're cooked in olive or similar quality oils.) By the way, since unsaturated oils like olive oil break down eventually, even at room temperature, no oil has a shelf life longer than a few months once it's opened. After such time the oil will be rancid, although undetectable by smell.

The omega-3 essential fatty acids are worthy of extra attention. These are oils found in nuts and seeds like flax and chia, as well as fish. While I wouldn't necessarily consider these fatty acids "essential," they do have great nutritive value. Omega-3 oils can lower cholesterol and are also blood thinning which naturally can be good for many of us. But again, like all other unsaturated fats, heating these oils destroys the health-producing effects. This is part of why you don't want to overcook fish. It's also why roasted nuts and seeds—as opposed to raw—aren't exactly healthy. Flaxseed oil can be a good product, but the raw seed as a whole food is how you get those omega-3s as fresh as possible. With fish oil products, there is a lot of debate as to whether they truly retain any beneficial value since the processing involves heat and oxygen. The data pertaining to the fatty acids being preserved for the sake of a long shelf-life is weak, and I believe the whole fish to be the superior option.

If you want to cook with oil, then it's important to use oils that are *saturated* fats which are more heat stable: butter or ghee (oil extracted from butter that is less likely to burn) or coconut oil for example. Ghee made from butter is completely heat stable making it perfect for any high-heat cooking. Ghee has been in the Ayurvedic diet of India for many years and is generally available at any natural food store. Coconut oil deserves special attention as well as a place in every kitchen pantry. In addition to being very heat stable, it has a healing effect on the thyroid. If you suspect that you're overweight due in part to a suppressed thyroid, then try taking raw, cold pressed, organic coconut oil (not palm oil which is unhealthy). It may sound counterintuitive that a saturated fat such as coconut can help with weight loss, but it can. Try it for yourself. Take one tablespoon daily in a smoothie or melt it into warm foods. Another benefit is that saturated fat like coconut lubricates the joints and bowels, helping them both to move a little better. Also the brain is *made* of saturated fat, making a supply of it important for the maintenance and regeneration of vital brain tissues.

Okay, I know what you must be thinking. Saturated fat? *Butter? Really?* Sure, it might be eyebrow-raising, but trust me. The key with saturated fats is moderation. Too much saturated fat will raise your cholesterol (even cholesterol-free oil like coconut oil). But is a tablespoon a day of these oils going to raise your cholesterol? Most likely not.

Animal Fats

A lot of questions that people seem to have about fats center on animal fats in particular. So let's consider a few of these.

Meats. Meats such as beef and chicken should represent only a small part of one's diet, if any part at all. These saturated fats can increase cholesterol and set a chain reaction towards heart disease and weight gain. The leaner (and less frequent) of these products the better. (Later in the book, we'll discuss animal protein.)

Eggs. Bad for you, right? Actually, no. Eggs can be an excellent food. Sure, they're high in cholesterol, but it's not a cholesterol that raises yours. There is saturated fat in eggs, but only to the tune of less than one gram per egg.

Dairy. This is a tradeoff. For protein and fat, milk isn't bad in moderation, but its main drawback is the presence of lactose (milk sugar) which is mucous-forming, making milk a little bit of a challenge for the body to digest. Yogurt's a little better than milk in this regard because the friendly bacteria partially break down the lactose making it more digestible. Note: stay away from pre-sweetened yogurt, which unfortunately represents ninety-percent of yogurts on the market. Most of them used processed sugar. Even the ones that brag about having real fruit still add extra sugar. Go with unsweetened yogurt, and then add the elite sweetener of your choice which we'll talk about more in the next chapter. Raw, unpasteurized dairy is growing in popularity because the idea is that it's less mucous-forming from maintaining the original enzymes which help digest the lactose.

If you do drink milk, it's best to go with skim milk, right? Wrong. The whole low-fat dairy thing has been problematic. Two-percent and skim milk should just be called what they are: lactose concentrate. They're hard to digest and a big part of why lactose sensitivity is becoming more common. Our bodies are rebelling. If you wish to have milk, then drink whole milk—just less of it. And you'll drink less of it because it'll satisfy much quicker than the milk sugar stuff.

Better still, make your own milk! If you have a high-powered blender (a fantastic investment), here's an easy alternative for milk: blend raw hemp seeds with water. Voila! No straining necessary. Add in a sprinkle of coconut sugar and cinnamon. This works well poured on unsweetened, flour-free cereals or as a creamer in smoothies. Homemade almond milk, while more labor intensive, is terrific, too. Boxed almond or soy or other nut milks in the store are less than ideal. Like all nuts and seeds, these are unsaturated oils that go rancid once heated and then packaged. Plus, these milks are often augmented with binders and thickeners to keep the water and oils from separating. Just more food processing that you don't need.

Bottom line: integrate healthy fats into your diet with primarily plant foods. Remember that the right fats can satisfy your appetite, thus helping to steer you clear from the processed carbs and sugars that everybody's been overeating due to the lack of satiation from the low-fat diet. Add a little cold-pressed olive oil to your salad and cook with butter, ghee, or coconut oil. (For more ideas, check out the recipes in the back.) In the realm of snack foods like chips and crackers, more and more products are becoming available that are made with temperature-stable oils, like coconut. Just be a conscious ingredient reader because the oils used have a tremendous influence! Even better, eat more raw (unroasted) nuts and seeds. The nutritive elites are pumpkin seeds, chia seeds, flax seeds, sesame seeds, and almonds. Walnuts, macadamia nuts, Brazil nuts, pistachios, and sunflower seeds have some nutritive value, too. Peanuts and cashews, though popular, aren't of much nutritive quality.

Okay, now that we've demystified fats, let's see if we can do the same with another hugely important topic: sugar.

THREE

How to Make Sugar Your Ally

As with fats, when it comes to sugar and health, the news isn't all bad. But the truth is, with sugar there's a huge amount of conflicting information out there as to what truly qualifies as "healthy." It's a vital question that is not taken seriously enough and, in fact, largely unanswered. So let's nail down the essential facts and the how-to's on how to get your sugar intake on the right track for truly enhancing your health—for both the body *and* mind. At first, applying this information to your diet may not be easy, but I promise it's not too difficult either, especially when you have the facts at hand! Believe that you can do this, and I'm confident you can. So, let's jump in and start with the upside of the topic.

The Drum Roll...

Sugar is important for our health! It's fuel— aka glucose. And a big reason it's important is that it's fuel that is quickly available to the body. While complex carbohydrates and fats can take hours to break down into fuel, sugar is put to use almost instantly. Now for the bad news. As a society, we've gone *way* down the wrong path with sugar. The sugar most people are ingesting today is refined sugar. This kind of sugar creates a scary amount of wear and tear on the body.

19

The Proof is in the Over-Sweetened Pudding

The seriousness of this state of affairs can't be overstated. Sugar, as it's found in many foods these days, is much worse than people think. Since it's so prevalent, most people just take the presence of sugar without concern for how harmful it really can be. The fact is, modern media have done an extraordinary job of making sugar look innocent. Showing attractive looking people drinking soda is deceitful irony.

Reality Check

The weakening effect sugar has on the body really deserves a book of its own. The data is abundant, and very real. Do an online search yourself. Let's spotlight a few of the most common detriments. Obesity—stuffing fat cells with high-glycemic calories is the body's natural defense to remedy the dangers of spiking blood sugar levels, from which come...diabetes—the body's intelligence with managing insulin levels can essentially be wiped out by sugar. Cancer—sad but true, processed sugar speeds the production of mutated cells. Osteoporosis—the body attempts to remedy the extreme acid-forming nature of sugar with calcium, and, yup, it's the precious calcium that comprises our bones. Digestive disorders—growth of fungus that can cause holes in the intestines? Ew, who wants that?! Numerous emotional and behavioral issues (especially with children) have clinically been linked to sugar. As for other vitally important mechanisms of the body such as hormone balance, the immune system, and the neurological system, they can all be compromised by processed sugar. And the familiar energy-crash that sugar creates essentially reflects all of the above maladies, making sugar a life-force depressant. This is a reflection of the simple fact that sugar makes the body weaker, thus more susceptible to disease.

What it is that Makes All of this Difficult? (And the Solution)

The big challenge in all of this is that processed sugar is in seemingly everything. You'll even find it in all those "natural" foods, such as cereal, crackers, yogurt, baked goods, and all the "low-fat" snacks—aisle after aisle of them and, sad to say, even at your natural food store. Even worse are the sweetened packaged drinks such as soda, energy drinks, sport drinks, and bottled tea. The manufacturers of these foods and drinks are clever, though. You won't necessarily find the word "sugar" in the ingredients. What you'll see instead is something like "evaporated cane juice." What's evaporated cane juice? You guessed it: sugar.

What really seals the deal on qualifying sugar as disastrous is the simple fact that it's chemically addictive. The common thought is *no, not for me*, but it's true, and there's no way around it. If you have sugar more than occasionally, I *dare* you to quit 100-percent cold-turkey. A few days into it, tell me you're not feeling an intense craving. Just a heads up: withdrawal symptoms, such as fatigue and headaches, are likely to come with it. Essentially the liver, kidneys, and the gastrointestinal system are detoxing. (If you take this dare, by the way, this would be a great time to detox your pantry, too, by tossing out all processed sugar.) In most cases, the sugar detox runs its course in about two weeks. At the end of it, it's likely you'll never want to go back. That's your body's wisdom kicking in now that the sugar spell is broken!

The Good News

Okay, with all that said, let's revisit the good news. Then we'll find a way to overcome the bad news. Your body needs sugar, so let's give it sugar. Let's feed that sweet tooth of yours. We all have one. It's a law of human biology. But let's be smart about how we do it. A craving for sweets can be friend or foe. We don't need to give up sugar; we just need to use the right sugar—the elite sugar. It's about getting the sugars that come with benefits. We're talking *nutrients*—vitamins, minerals, antioxidants, and enzymes!

The Remedy

Where can we find elite, truly healthy sugar? That's easy: the produce section of your local grocery store. Fruit! This is where the elite sugar hangs out. Matching your sugar intake primarily with fruit is the fundamental solution behind getting the whole dilemma resolved! It's *fruit* that's the key ally for keeping that sweet tooth of yours happy, helping you steer clear of the processed stuff that makes everything weaker in the name of entertaining taste-buds.

There's a bit more to it though. First, not all fruit sugar is the same. Some fruits are indeed more health enhancing than others. Let's cut to the chase and identify the elites. The elite fruits are primarily berries. We're talking blackberries, strawberries, and blueberries, to name a few of the most common ones. Color is often reflective of a plant food's nutrients. Another great thing about berries is that they're generally low-glycemic. This means the sugar in these foods is slower burning and therefore gentler in raising and lowering your blood sugar. Processed sugar, by contrast, is extremely high-glycemic, quickly burning and sending your blood sugar up and down and all over the place.

There are some higher glycemic fruits, too. Tropical fruits like bananas, pineapple, papaya, and mango are high glycemic, relative to berries. But that doesn't necessarily make them bad. These tropical fruits still have nutrients and are in no way comparable to the processed stuff. In moderation, they can serve an excellent role. I find them to be perfect as sweeteners in smoothies. Somewhere in the middle of the glycemic scale you have the other fruits you might think of: pears, apples, oranges, watermelon, etc. They're all good for you.

The key here is that having fruit in the morning and again in the afternoon will keep your sweet tooth happy throughout the day. You'll be a lot less tempted to grab a donut from the break room or order a sugar-filled dessert at lunch. We all know the problem with trying to have just one cookie or one small slice of chocolate cake. Generally, the struggle for discipline turns into a landslide of overdoing it. With whole unprocessed fruits, it's hard to overdo it and the margin for error is wide, especially with those berries. But many fruits, like anything in life, require some degree of moderation. What qualifies as moderation is different for everyone, but I believe in our body's instincts when it comes to healthy unprocessed plant foods. Sure, I wouldn't necessarily recommend eating three bananas, but when we're talking sugar, it's more a matter of quality than quantity. (Of course the same goes for complex carbs, protein, and fat too.) Between the sugar in fruit and processed sugar, there's no comparison. When it comes to whole foods like fruit, we have an instinctive sense as to what the right amount is, a sense that unfortunately becomes distorted by processed sugar that is nowhere in the scope of the body's instincts. Thankfully we're on our way to restoring this wisdom of the body!

What about fruit juice? Well, the whole fruit is always better. Juicing eliminates some of the nutrients and all of the fiber. Beware of the common pasteurized juices at your supermarket, which is most of them. And don't be fooled by the bottled "superfood" or "health" drinks with overdosing amounts of pasteurized fruit juice. Besides the high sugar content, the pasteurization process in and of itself isn't good. Pasteurization is necessary for lengthening shelf life; these refrigerated and bottled juices might be on the shelf for weeks or even months. Without pasteurization, they'll ferment in just a few days. Pasteurization means essentially cooking the juice, torching the nutrients, and eliminating the otherwise awesome health benefits. If you're going to drink fruit juice, stick with raw and fresh-pressed juice. Even still, fruit juice of any sort without the original fiber of the whole fruit is going to give you a burst of glucose. So unless you become physically active soon after drinking it, your body will store that fuel someplace that will be less than flattering. Thus my preference for the whole fruit.

Among fruit drinks, my top pick is a smoothie using whole fruit with its fiber and nutrients—an especially great choice in the morning. You need fuel first thing in the morning, and your body will respond especially well to a smoothie which is easy to digest as the gastrointestinal system is just revving up. Here's my favorite: a frozen banana in the blender with pure water and a round tablespoon of raw almond butter. This is a perfect opportunity to use Infinity Greens. The energy from the fruit and superfoods will be sustained by the healthy fats from the almond butter for a slow burn that will last for hours. A blend like this is ideal because the balance between sugar, fat, and protein will smooth out the natural ups and downs of your blood sugar. Fruit sugars are infinitely better than processed sugars, but they still affect the level of your blood sugar. What goes up must come down. But a well-balanced smoothie with the right fruit, protein, and fat together can be the perfect low-calorie, energy-sustaining, nutrient-dense breakfast!

The Right Combination

As with smoothies, here's a great thing to do with fruit: combine it with protein-fats, like nuts and seeds. As we talked about, sugar produces the quick energy, and protein-fat sustains it. Think up your own combinations. A banana split? Hmm...think a little harder. How about strawberries and yogurt? Much better. Raw sprouted almonds and prunes? Perfect. Apples and raw almond butter? Now you're talking. Of course fruits don't necessarily have to be eaten with anything else (and are still great to have by themselves), but when combined with protein-fats, you'll satisfy your appetite much longer. Note: it's better for fruits *not* to be combined with other complex carbohydrates, like grains and vegetables. This combination produces fermentation in the gastrointestinal system which isn't good if done on a routine basis. Once in awhile, no big deal. Best to have your fruit first, which digests in just minutes, then the bigger meal shortly after.

Now let's revisit the processed sugars. Some actually aren't so bad. Here are my top picks. Maple syrup. We're talking tree sap, not the Aunt Jemima kind. She may have been a sweet lady, but her syrup is little more than high-fructose corn syrup which is in the same category as white sugar and is no better than terrible. High fructose corn syrup is especially common in bottled drinks. It's a high-consequence processed sugar, particularly with obesity, and ironically makes up a significant portion of the average American's daily calories. Real maple syrup on the other hand is rich in minerals and is perfectly fine when used in moderation. Raw honey has my golden stamp of approval. Unheated honey has an immune boosting, health-enhancing value of its own.

Coconut sugar is up there, too. Like maple syrup, coconut sugar is tree sap, only dried. It's mineral-rich and low-glycemic. The brilliance of coconut sugar is you can use it gram for gram in recipes where you would otherwise use processed sugar, only the flavor is *better* and the calories are *fewer.*

Other middle of the road processed sugars include brown rice syrup, yacon syrup, and lucuma berry syrup. The once-popular agave nectar and sucanat are further down the totem pole. Sucanat is a whole cane sweetener that retains the original molasses, making it better than processed sugar. Molasses separated from cane sugar is actually mineral-rich and is the one perk of cane plants. Sucanat isn't as popular as processed sugar, because not everyone is fond of the taste of molasses. Plus it's triple the cost of white sugar. Although it's better, it's still high-glycemic and not exactly health-forming. What about brown sugar? Brown sugar has a sprits of molasses added back to the processed sugar, making it no better than white sugar.

Other Sweeteners

If you're looking for a zero-calorie sweetener, try stevia (not Splenda). Stevia is a natural leaf with a sweet flavor and no unhealthy qualities. I recommend green stevia powder which is simply the whole ground-up stevia leaf. The common bleached stevia with maltodextrin isn't necessarily bad, but the less processed product is always better.

What about Aspartame? Marketed as NutraSweet, Equal, and other innocent names, it's been shown to be chemically addictive. During my years of teaching nutrition at the *Ashram Health Retreat*, I would always see the diet soda drinkers having a rough detox experience. Diet soda is really among the worst things you can put into your body. Xylitol: beware of it as a sweetener. This is sugar alcohol extracted from corn through an award-winning amount of processing. It really shouldn't be ingested for the simple reason that it draws water from the body into the intestines which is obviously not good for more than just a few reasons. Same goes with sorbitol.

A Note about Chocolate

As I would be talking about sugar in my nutrition classes, there would inevitably be someone wearing a look of mild despair who would ask for my thoughts about chocolate. Well cacao in chocolate products can actually have beneficial nutritive properties, including the presence of soluble fiber, magnesium, healthy saturated fats, and antioxidants. Theobroma in chocolate *is* a stimulant, making it something to enjoy only in moderation, but all in all, the right chocolate can be a healthy food. This would always make everyone in the class breathe a sigh of relief. But are we talking about chocolate cake here? Nope, definitely not. The wear and tear from the over-saturation of sugar and flour unquestionably outweigh the pluses of the chocolate. And sorry, we're not talking chocolate candy bars, either. Your average chocolate candy bar, loaded with sugar, hypnotizes those taste buds, making you eat the whole thing, and more. In dark chocolate (labeled eighty-five percent cacao), a one ounce serving has only three grams of sugar. This level of sugar almost qualifies more as a "flavor" than a sweetener, making it less of a big deal in my opinion. However, if you search enough at your local natural food store, you can likely find dark chocolate sweetened with coconut sugar or honey. Now we're talking.

Another plus of dark chocolate is that it satisfies that sweet-tooth craving, even with a very small amount. One ounce generally does the trick. Better than dark chocolate is the original chocolate bean. These are generally available at your local store crushed up into nibs. With most high-quality brands, the nibs are raw and unheated, preserving the antioxidant value. There are plenty of ways to enjoy them, like in oatmeal or a smoothie. Try them with dried fruit. Even by themselves, I think nibs are tasty. Raw unsweetened chocolate is also available in the form of powder. Why not create your own chocolate dessert using only premium ingredients? I've shared a few in the Appendix.

Making it Easy

Your body needs natural sugar and now you know the right places to find it. First thing tomorrow, make yourself a smoothie. Throw the glazed donut away, along with the "natural" junk food. Have some of that healthy sugar in the afternoon, too. Feed your sweet tooth with nutrient rich fruit. Why not have a pear, a slice of watermelon, or a peach? How about berries with lunch? So many options! Eliminate the sugar-filled desserts. Forego sweet drinks—soda, energy drinks, bottled fruit juices, pre-packaged smoothies, sweetened teas, etc.

Here is my humble yet hearty recommendation: go for the two-week challenge and completely cut processed sugar from your diet. If weight loss is at all a priority for you then this is an especially important thing to do (this will only be one benefit among many). And again, detox that pantry. Throw everything away that has processed sugar or "evaporated cane juice" or "corn syrup." And while you're at it, toss the stuff with artificial sweeteners, too. Please remember my fair warning: processed sugar (and Aspartame) is addictive! That means that giving it up won't be easy. It'll take some discipline, but hang in there. It will be among the best things you do for yourself. After the two weeks, any urge you have for processed sugar will likely be gone, or at least substantially reduced. Life is simply better without it, for both the body *and* mind. Trust me. And following our protocol of replacing processed sweets with the goodness of sweets from fruit (have two to four pieces a day) will make the whole thing very doable. I promise you'll be glad you did this for yourself!

In addition to simply eating healthier, you'll discover something amazing. As with any healthy protocol, when you give your body what it truly wants and you begin to feel the benefits, you'll notice that you'll start to naturally gravitate towards those things that make you feel great. Don't be surprised if you don't find cake and ice cream as appealing as you used to. Once you're on the healthy, energetic path, you'll find it relatively easy to stay on it. Such is the brilliance of your body's natural intelligence. Pretty sweet, eh?

FOUR

Carbs Demystified

There's a lot of confusion about carbohydrates. We hear about simple and complex carbs, but what's the difference? What do these terms even mean? In its most basic sense, a carbohydrate is a compound of carbon, hydrogen, and oxygen. Carbohydrates are present in the foods we eat, and our body breaks them down into glucose that can then be used as energy.

Simple Versus Complex

Simple carbohydrates are, essentially, just sugar. Like we talked about, they're found in the average diet, predominantly as processed sugar, such as cane sugar and high fructose corn syrup. Most of the simple carbohydrates in the modern diet are unhealthy, although there are exceptions, including honey and pure maple syrup (in moderation), as we mentioned in the last chapter. Fresh-pressed (unpasteurized) fruit juice is essentially fructose or fruit sugar, thus making it a simple carbohydrate too.

Generally, complex carbohydrates are a combination of starch (chains of sugar) and fiber (non-caloric plant matter). This is why whole fruit, because of its fiber, is actually a complex carbohydrate, although it's often thought of as a simple carbohydrate because

29

of the sugar. Besides whole fruit, complex carbs include vegetables, beans, bread, pasta, and all grains such as oats, rye, quinoa, rice, millet, and wheat. Of course some complex carbohydrates are healthier than others. Essentially, the healthy complex carbohydrates are unprocessed plant foods and whole grains. As we'll discuss in a bit, these unprocessed complex carbohydrates give you the fiber and nutrients.

The Perils of Processed Foods

Okay, so let's talk first about the unhealthy complex carbs: *processed* complex carbohydrates. These are among the greatest culprits of weight gain (and many other health problems) today. Most of the processed complex carbohydrates are basically grains that have been robbed of their fiber and nutrients, becoming concentrates of starch. Examples of foods high in processed carbs include most cereal, most bread, pasta, crackers, chips, most baked foods (among the worst are the "low-fat" snack foods), and basically anything with flour. When flour is made, the grain is stripped of the fiber husk and pulverized into a fine powder, leaving nothing but the caloric starch. These foods are quite abundant, even at your natural food store, and, I dare say, make up the majority of products sold.

Here's the problem: what happens with these "calorie concentrates" is that they behave similarly to processed sugars. Because of their processed nature, they're digested quickly, causing an overdose of glucose that the body has no choice but to store as energy for later, which, you guessed it, is stored as fat. Yup, that's how it works. This is why processed foods, even in smaller amounts, are such major weight-gain foods. And they're extremely easy to overdo since, without the original fiber and nutrients, they don't satisfy the appetite. Even worse, the missing nutrients are actually needed for the food to be properly metabolized which are then borrowed from the body's reserves in order to do so. So, it's a triple whammy. They're fattening in and of themselves, depleting, and you eat more of them to boot. *Doh!* Even a small amount of processed food goes a long way—especially around the waist line.

Distressingly, these foods can be hard to get away from. For most people, their intake begins first thing in the morning with a seemingly innocent bowl of cereal. Some of the cereals in your grocery store appear to be healthy, but do you always remember to read the ingredients? The front of the box may say "natural," "organic," and "whole grain," but look at the side of the box. Most cereals, despite what they say on the front, have flour in them. Furthermore, they also have "evaporated cane juice" which, as you'll recall from earlier, is just straight-up processed sugar disguised by a natural-sounding name. Not good.

So, what can you use as a breakfast cereal instead? How about oatmeal? No, not instant oatmeal with sweeteners. Instead, use whole rolled oats! (The "how-to"? Simply cook in water. If you add oil, remember to use a healthy, heat-stable option such as ghee, butter, or coconut oil. Once cooled to an eating temperature add raw nuts, seeds, and unsweetened yogurt. You can even get some of your healthy sugar with sliced berries and a drizzle of honey. Now that's a balanced breakfast!) If you want to stick with cereal, look for the brands that don't contain sugar or flour. There are a few out there. The Ezekiel brand cereal has my approval, since it constitutes only the whole-wheat berry. For bread, same thing—simply stay away from flour. Unfortunately, that's ninety-five percent of the breads on the market. Again, you can look for the Ezekiel brand since they produce better options for bread and tortillas too. Manna Bread is a decent brand as well. The main factor is these options are flourless. Lucky for you, there's an entire section of recipes in the back of this very book that will make avoiding processed flour easy.

Gluten

While we're talking about the perils of processed foods, let's talk about something that seems to be attracting a lot of attention lately:

gluten. We hear a lot about it, but few of us know what the issue really is. Is gluten bad for us? What does it do? And just what the heck is it anyway?

To put it simply, gluten is the protein component in grains such as wheat, spelt, and barley. And it's now in almost everything we eat. Think about the popular foods most Americans consume throughout any given day: cereal (cold or hot), toast, pastries, tortillas, pizza, crackers, cookies, energy bars, breaded meats, sandwiches, pastas, soy sauce, salad dressing, thick sauces, soups and soup bases, beer, desserts...and more bread! This means we're constantly eating gluten.

The problem with gluten is that it's hard to digest. Our bodies simply haven't adapted to today's prevalence of so much gluten in our foods. We can handle it in moderation, but we've gone way beyond *that*. With a high intake of gluten, the digestive system has to work harder and, over time, this means wear and tear. And this is why many of us are becoming gluten-sensitive.

Some people are actually gluten-intolerant, so even a little is problematic. People living with celiac disease fall into this category. Celiac disease is a rare autoimmune disorder and we'll look more closely at some autoimmune disorders later in the book. For now, we'll focus on gluten sensitivity.

Specifically, how do we reduce gluten? Mostly by being aware of its presence. The biggest culprit is wheat flour. Think of wheat flour as gluten concentrate. We just finished talking about why processed foods are unhealthy and gluten in wheat flour gives us just one more reason.

I know it's hard to keep away from wheat flour since it's everywhere, but there are alternatives. Unprocessed options can include rice, quinoa, and corn. For breads, don't forget the sprouted grain breads we mentioned above. They're flourless. One-hundred-percent rye breads are a good bet, too. But I mean one-hundred percent. All grocery stores sell "rye" bread, but most often it's *flavored* with rye with wheat still as the main ingredient.

Be careful not to rely on all the "gluten-free" (GF) foods that are out there nowadays. GF baked snacks have become very popular, but a lot of them just use other processed starchy grains instead of wheat. And so you're just substituting one kind of processed food for another!

Listen to your body. If you're finding that you have some reactions to wheat products, try cutting out wheat flour or at least significantly reducing your intake. Instead of having those rolls with dinner, just steam up a bit of quinoa or rice.

For any kind of food sensitivity, your goal should be to strengthen your digestive system, one of the major pillars of good health! You and your digestive system should be working together, not against each other. We'll delve into this subject later in the book.

The Key

The key is simply to remember this: more unprocessed foods. Simple? Yes, but not necessarily easy. However, as we discussed earlier, the processed grains without the original fiber and nutrients are merely unsatisfying, fast-digesting calories. Bottom line: enhance your diet to include more of the best unprocessed complex carbohydrates (vegetables, whole fruit, whole grains). This will be reflected in anyone's health, especially long-term. An added bonus is that your days of calorie-counting will be pretty much over. This is because it's near impossible to overeat low-calorie-density foods such as broccoli. Incorporating more of *these* foods into our diets enables us to much more easily reduce our calories, if need be (which applies to many of us).

What's more is that fibrous foods are good for the digestive tract and have countless other health benefits. It's also worth mentioning that green foods deserve a sturdy presence in our diet: broccoli, cabbage, kale, spinach, mustard greens, collard greens, and green beans, to name a few. These have the most fiber and nutrients relative to the starch content. These are the foods that satiate the appetite the most per calorie. We will take a further look into green foods in Chapter 6.

I should also note that among the complex carbs, white potatoes aren't so great since they have loads of starch and very little fiber and nutrition (not to mention that they are often dressed up with loads of sour cream and bacon bits. Ha!). Sweet potatoes, at the *other* end of the spectrum, are awesome.

As for grains, my first pick is rice. And white rice, specifically. It's been in the human diet for thousands of years in many places around the world and is something our digestion is perfectly adapted to. Brown rice is good too, but really has only become popular in recent years here in the western world. Sure, brown rice has fiber but it's also much harder to digest than white rice. The better philosophy is to get your fiber from the vegetables cooked *with* the rice. Quinoa is great too. However, it is a food that doesn't always digest perfectly for everyone. You'll have to try it to see for yourself. Millet and amaranth are cool, but are also not the easiest to digest either. Beans and lentils have complex carbohydrates *and* protein and are both excellent foods.

You may be happy to know another food that gets my stamp of approval is popcorn. But only air-popped, or stovetop cooked with heat-stable coconut oil. Popcorn at the movie theater definitely does not fall into this category. Nor does the packaged popcorn that's already popped, since the oils will be rancid. And need I say anything about microwave popcorn? Home-cooked unadulterated popcorn is great. Add a little Celtic sea salt if you wish. It's high in insoluble fiber, and low in calories per volume, making it pretty hard to overdo.

Coming full circle, I understand that a complete dietary overhaul for some of us may be a bit overwhelming. Cereals and breads and snacks have become dietary staples for many of us. But if you make a conscious effort to start substituting with healthier, unprocessed foods, you'll notice a funny thing start to happen. The processed junk will actually begin to seem unappetizing to you.

Very truthfully, processed foods like bread, crackers, chips, and other snack foods have become totally and completely repulsive to me. Why? Because of something we talked about earlier: the body recognizes nutrient-rich foods and, if given a steady supply, will naturally gravitate towards the good stuff and away from all the junk. It's true. Believe me. I saw it countless times during my years at the Ashram. During the course of their time there, guests would develop an improved taste for good, healthy, nutritious, lower-calorie, natural, unprocessed food. They'd come back a year later looking and feeling like different people. The difference? They successfully incorporated the Ashram dietary principles into their lives. Furthermore, they reported that it was less than difficult for them to do so and that they had no interest in going back to their old dietary ways. Try it yourself and see if the same thing doesn't happen to you. I have a hunch your body's instinctual wisdom may just tip the scale in your favor.

Okay, we've talked about fats, we've talked about sugars, we've talked about carbs. Let's turn our attention now to something every bit as important: protein.

FIVE

The Protein Solution

Why is protein worth special attention? Because protein is the primary building block of muscle, ligaments, cartilage, vital organs, and essentially every cell in the body. You really *are* what you eat! That's why. So I say let's use the finest building blocks that we have available.

Unfortunately, as a species, we've made things complicated for ourselves, and our intake of protein is now a matter that desperately needs a shift. First, consider that for thousands of years, since our days as hunter-gatherers, our major source of protein has been animals. Before the advent of today's food distribution, people could only eat what they could find in their immediate surroundings. Especially in the winter months, that could mean just meat and potatoes. But from our ancestors' simpler days of hunting wild animals for food, we've gone down a different path. Today, our Western diet is plagued by poor quality meat—and lots of it!

Moreover, very definite data now exist that show a connection between the consumption of today's animal protein and cancer and heart disease. Processed beef and pork have been newly classified by the World Health Organization as Level One carcinogens. That's the same as cigarettes! Eek! Isn't that nuts? And few people even know about this. Let's consider this a red flag.

37

The Flaws of Modern Day Protein

The days of low-grade beef, pork, and chicken have caught up with us. This meat is definitely protein, but it's the wear and tear on our overall health that comes with it that needs our attention.

Part of the problem is the type of saturated fats that come with animal protein. *These* are the fats that very definitely can raise unhealthy cholesterol—a separate book entirely. Even with the low-fat meat products, a little lard can go a long way, and not in our favor! I feel that the fats in meat are actually a big part of why we crave them. Ah, the smell of bacon many of us mysteriously appreciate. Because cutting back on *all* fat in our overall diet is a dominant theme, we eventually cave in and get our fat fix from animal products. But satisfying our need for fats with animal lard is akin to satisfying the sweet tooth with processed sugar instead of fruit.

Another consideration: meats are acid-forming. Quick lesson: our bodies seek to strike a healthy acid-alkaline chemistry that's affected mostly by the foods we eat. All animal protein makes the body acidic (as does processed sugar, interestingly enough). An "acidic" internal environment ultimately translates into a decrease of calcium in bones and an increase of inflammation in tissues causing reduced blood flow, which ultimately translates to a weaker body that simply ages faster than it regenerates. And in case you're wondering, chicken is just as acid-forming as red meat, so you're not really doing your body any favors by sticking with just "white" low-fat meat.

Additionally, metabolic waste from regular animal protein can accumulate over time in the gastrointestinal system. An eight-ounce steak isn't eight ounces of protein, after all. A lot of it is indigestible animal matter which can build up in your large intestine and colon, slowly but surely weakening your digestive system, a vital pillar of your health.

Also, ever notice you're tired after eating meat? Even just a chicken salad? This is because it actually takes a lot of work for your body to break it down to extract the protein. So if you do have any animal protein in your diet, you might want to consider limiting it as a dinner food.

But what about Fish?

I believe having a little fish in your diet can offer some overall benefits. Certain fish can be excellent food nutritionally and a far superior option to other meat products. One of the reasons is ease of digestibility. And like we talked about in Chapter 2, the other advantage of fish is the quality of fat. Remember fish oils contain omega-3 fatty acids which have the exact opposite effect of the fats in other meat products. These fats actually *reduce* unhealthy cholesterol.

With all fish, be sure to go with wild-caught and avoid farm-raised fish. A lot of the fish today are farm-raised where the fish are crowded together, producing unclean conditions that require major amounts of antibiotics and pesticides. Even salmon labeled as "Atlantic salmon" is, more likely than not, farm-raised. If salmon or any fish are wild-caught it will clearly say "wild-caught" on the label.

If fish is a regular part of your diet, it's also important to be aware of fish that are known to be high in mercury as well as other harmful contaminants. Fish repeatedly testing high in mercury include tuna (especially albacore, ahi, and yellowfin tuna; skipjack tuna is okay), swordfish, shark, grouper, marlin, and mackerel. I suggest avoiding these entirely. Stick with the options tested to be low-mercury. These include salmon, trout, tilapia, sole, and most smaller fish. Other seafood like shrimp, oysters, and scallops tend to be okay too. In general, it's the large predatory fish that have toxic levels of mercury, even with freshwater fish.

B12

If there's one nutrient that stubbornly keeps meat relevant in the conversation, it's this one. Why? Because—unfortunately—B12 isn't found in plant foods. B12 is super important for maintaining healthy nerve cells, producing red blood cells, and serving a number of other vitally important tasks. So what to do? One decent source of vegetarian B12 are eggs, the nutritional value of which we talked about in Chapter 2. Dairy is also a fair solution, which we'll cover in more detail later in the book. Yogurt, cheese, and milk all have small amounts of B12. Certain fish, like salmon, are an excellent source of B12, too.

But what if your system is sensitive to eggs and dairy, or you're living a vegetarian lifestyle? In this case it's wise to consider a B12 supplement. Bear in mind that I typically don't endorse anything that's made in a laboratory and is not from real food. But lab-formulated B12 is one exception and is definitely better than no B12 at all. And where should you look for B12 supplements? Let's start with where you shouldn't look. So-called fortified foods (like fortified cereals and breads and soy products) commonly use a synthetic B12 called cyanocobalamin, which is known to be mildly toxic with long-term use. Not so good. A better alternative is methylcobalamin B12. This B12 is available by injection, sublingual liquid, patches, and capsules at your local natural food store.

Something to remember, by the way, is that B12 can be stored in the body for years. So if you're a newly-converted vegetarian or vegan, you'll be fine for a while. But down the road, you're going to need a plan for making sure you're getting a sufficient quantity of B12.

Note: an important solution for preventing B12 deficiency is to avoid a lifestyle that depletes it. Get rid of the processed foods, limit your intake of caffeine, alcohol, and tobacco (preferably eliminate)—all of which can very definitely drain your body of B12. As always, your health is largely defined by your lifestyle, especially over time! Have confidence in your instincts and exercise your discipline to make health-enhancing lifestyle choices.

By the way, besides B12, I often get asked about two other nutrients found in meat; namely, iron and zinc. Where besides meat can these be found? Lots of places! High iron plant foods include edamame, tempeh, lentils, cooked spinach, chick peas, chard, pumpkin seeds, figs, and blue-green algae like spirulina. Zinc can be found in watermelon seeds, cooked spinach, avocado, asparagus, broccoli, chard, and collard greens. There. Easy enough.

As for the Vegetarian Lifestyle

If you've been thinking of trying a vegetarian diet, I say why not? Today, with the large variety of foods we have available year round, we can in most cases get all the protein and nutrients the body needs without animal protein. Or getting your animal protein exclusively from fish can be an excellent option too.

I feel it's worth sharing that for two years I was on the "Paleo" diet, a popular diet that is quite high in animal protein. I kept to the better quality options like bison, elk, venison, and meats of similar nature. These meats are definitely better alternatives to the more common meats like beef and pork. Even still, at the end of the day, I found that the Paleo diet yielded much less energy and sense of life-force than a diet without these animal products.

If you continue to have meat as a regular part of your diet, it's still good to take breaks! Going a couple weeks without meat, adding more plant foods in place of it, allows your body to go through its important cleansing cycles.

While we're on the subject, I should say this. Many people take an ethical position on the eating of meat. In case you're wondering, my role here is nutrition and so I'm going to keep within those bounds. I'll leave the ethical question to each individual reader. Nevertheless, I do feel that a primarily plant-based diet with the right foods is the superior option for overall health.

Where to Find the Protein

Okay, so where can you find the plant foods high in protein, the plant foods you'll need in order to compensate for cutting back (or maybe even eliminating) meat? Easy. High protein vegetarian foods include raw nuts and seeds, avocados, beans, edamame, eggs, and dairy. Protein supplements can also play an excellent role here. But beware of whey or soy based protein. They're culprits of constipation, like eating glue. Hemp and rice protein get my stamp of approval.

Note: don't make *this* mistake frequently made by people cutting back on meat: replacing meat with pasta, bread, processed grains, and other starchy foods. You're looking for protein, not tons of starch! As for my recommendation of how many grams of protein to have per day, I'd put this in the same category as counting calories. Unnecessary. Follow the suggestions above and there's really not a margin of error you need to be given since your body's tastes and instincts will be allowed to do the job they were born to do.

Okay, so here's the big picture. The Western world eats way too much animal protein (especially the worst kind!). Kind of like unhealthy sugar. But in the end, it comes down to a lifestyle choice. And who wants a lifestyle that includes foods that slowly make you weaker, little by little chipping away at your body's overall health and life force?

It doesn't help, of course, that beef, pork, and chicken are so prevalent. It's the main part of most entrees in most restaurants! And few people know how high-impact this part of their diet can be. But now you do. If you're starting to become more and more sold on the healthier proteins, then fantastic. If we'd collectively cut back on the common low-quality meats, we'd be doing something extraordinary for ourselves (not to mention the planet!). Yes, we have the hunter-gatherer in our genes, but we also have the option to live a lot healthier than our ancestors did— and longer too. And as we've seen, because of today's variety and availability of plant food and healthier protein, this can be easy to do.

SIX

The Critical Element in Green Foods

Quick review. So far, we've talked about fats, sugar, starch, and protein. We've talked about some things you should be eating, and we've talked about some things you shouldn't be eating. Mostly the latter. Now the time has come to start addressing the greatest high-impact foods of a healthy diet. Now it's time to talk about *greens*. Green foods deserve a chapter of their own for just their cleansing and restorative power alone. But there are a number of other reasons, too, as we'll soon see!

The Beauty of these Dual-Purpose Foods

When we're talking about greens, we're talking about foods like kale, arugula, chard, mustard greens, collard greens, parsley, cilantro, spinach, basil, broccoli, and blue-green algae. (*Algae?* Yup. We'll be talking about this subject shortly.) What makes these foods *vitally* important for a healthy diet? There are two reasons and one might surprise you. The first is obvious: green foods are rich in nutrients, especially the ones that help the body to maintain its youth and vitality.

43

But the second reason often gets overlooked. Green foods are essential for eliminating toxins from the body. And this is a bigger deal than you might realize. Think about it. Our bodies are bombarded with toxins every day, especially here in the twenty-first century. In the air we breathe, the water we drink, and the food we eat, we're exposed to impurities that people never had to worry about before. This is wear and tear enough. Add to it the normal everyday stresses from life itself, and you can readily see why the cleansing goodness of greens is so important to our diets and health. Quite simply, their impact is huge!

The Magic behind Greens

What specifically is it about greens that gives them the unmatched power to cleanse and restore our bodies from toxins? A little something you might remember from high school biology: *chlorophyll*. This is the magical element in green foods. (It's also what makes them green.) It's the chlorophyll itself that bonds to toxins in your body, enabling them to be eliminated via the gastrointestinal system. This is indeed a critical means of avoiding the buildup of toxins in your body. Consider that it's the buildup of toxins that's a primary instigator of disease, as well as aging.

The Weight-Loss Connection is Worthy of Mention

Interestingly, bodily fat attempts to protect the body from toxins, too. This is a little-known reason that losing fat can be so challenging. Collectively, fat cells absorb toxins from the bloodstream for the sake of protecting vital organs. It's a temporary form of self defense. The problem is that when the body needs to later burn this "toxic fat-fuel" for energy, it becomes reluctant to do so because that means toxins would go back into the bloodstream (which would then cause wear and tear on other things in the body). So let green foods fulfill their vital role of removing toxins, making way for fat to be burned as fuel.

Additionally, green foods are very low calorie, and this factor coupled with the nutrient density makes way for satisfying the appetite with fewer calories. Naturally, this enhances the potential for weight loss (which, statistically, should be a priority for more people than not). Fat reduction: yet another reason for adding more green foods to your diet!

And vitamin K! Kale, spinach, chard, collard greens, mustard greens and broccoli are the most vitamin K rich foods. Vitamin K is important for a lot of reasons, but the most critical is blood clotting and repair of damaged tissues in the body. Talk about a healing food!

Keep it Simple

So from a dietary standpoint, think "clean and green." Introduce more dark green foods into your diet to get your chlorophyll and vital nutrients. How about salads? Well, sure. But don't make the common mistake of fooling yourself into thinking a salad of lettuce with a couple of wedges of tomato covered with packaged salad dressing is going to do the trick. We're talking unadulterated *dark* greens. And keep it simple. Why not go hand to mouth? That's what I do. Grab a few large leaves of kale or chard or a couple handfuls of spinach or arugula or any other leafy greens and chow down. You can eat greens just as they are.

Personally, I find greens to be tasty (they most certainly don't taste bad) and see little reason to add anything to them. But if you want to toss a little homemade *healthy* salad dressing into the mix, have at it. Olive oil, lemon juice, sea salt, and cayenne. Simple. A tried and true classic. (Please don't even bother with the packaged salad dressings which are nothing more than unhealthy entertainment. What the heck is ranch dressing, anyway? Ever read the ingredients of those dressings? Straight up junk food! Even the "natural" ones.)

And then there's green sauce! This is one of my favorite recipes and one that we should all be making. You put the same salad dressing ingredients (olive oil, lemon juice, sea salt, and cayenne) into the blender with raw greens like spinach or kale. An advantage of this is it makes these foods easy to digest. At times, the coarser green foods can actually be a little hard for the body to break down. It's cellulose that gives plants their rigidity so they don't just flop over in the dirt. Blending them essentially breaks down the cellulose walls which makes them easy to digest *and* maintains the chlorophyll. This recipe tastes amazing and is brilliant as a sauce over other cooked foods, or as a dip. (See the Appendix.)

Cooked greens still provide all of the minerals, but it's good to keep in mind the chlorophyll will likely break down, depending on how heavily they are cooked. When greens are bright in color post-steaming, that means there's still chlorophyll. Cooking them, similar to blending, also breaks down the cellulose—another reason to mix it up between cooked and raw.

Another factor to consider is that green foods like kale, cabbage, broccoli, spinach, collard and mustard greens, when *raw*, and in large quantities, can actually have a mildly suppressive effect on the thyroid, which controls our metabolic rate. A weak thyroid is somewhat common. (The main culprit today is fried food and other cooked unsaturated oils that we talked about in Chapter 2. Processed soy products can do the same too.) Then again, some people have an overactive thyroid, so turning it down mildly with these green foods isn't necessarily bad. It's a matter of balance, having them both cooked *and* raw. Personally I cook my greens about half of the time. Steam them, sauté them, put 'em in soups. Again, you'll lose some of the chlorophyll, but when cooked (or blended), the minerals actually become more easily absorbable. For raw greens, have the majority of these as the "baby greens" that are softer, making them easier to digest.

As for how much green food to have in your daily diet, definitely more than just a sprits of greens on your sandwich. A simple and reliable gauge is the "large handful." This is another thing with which your instinctive wisdom can play an outstanding role. There's memory of green foods in our genes since these foods have been in the human diet for many thousands of years. So your body knows. Trust those instincts.

Algae

Even among the healthiest green foods, there's one group worthy of extra mention. Based on my nutrition research and experience, I rank algae at the top of the ladder of the most health enhancing foods. Interestingly, algae were the very first life on earth—beginning three and a half billion years ago. Essentially, algae are the ancient foundation of our food chain. It's fascinating that now we're turning back to the very first food on earth for nutritional support.

There are thousands of different algae, most of which can't be consumed. However, edible varieties of algae have been in the human diet as far back as recorded history will take us—and all over the world—except for the last few hundred years in the Western world. Only recently have we begun hearing a lot more about the nutritive attributes of algae. Why this recent interest? Because algae have the highest concentration of chlorophyll of any food you can name. This is what makes algae so green!

It's also worth mentioning that algae produce over sixty percent of the oxygen in our atmosphere and are the most powerful photosynthesizers on our planet, harnessing directly the energy of the sun. Sun plus water and minerals miraculously creates algae—then *poof!*—oxygen, which is among the more important elements of life, wouldn't you say? This magical process happens in the body as well. Algae oxygenate the blood which naturally has a tremendous impact on our energy and overall health, especially in conjunction with the chlorophyll.

The Trio

Among the different types of algae, it's Klamath algae, spirulina, and chlorella that have the most remarkable health forming qualities.

47

Numerous blind studies have proven the significant nutritive and restorative value of these algae. Here is a brief summary of what makes each of these three algae truly worthy of our attention.

Klamath algae is recognized for its extraordinary support of the nervous system. Klamath algae metabolizes nitrogen in the body which stimulates the production of more neurotransmitters in the brain. Neurotransmitters are the link that carries messages from the brain to the body and then from the body back to the brain. In addition, anecdotal reports consistently attribute Klamath algae consumption to an increase in mental alertness and memory retention.

Spirulina is among the few richest sources of beta-carotene, which is reputed to be an important anti-cancer antioxidant. Beta-carotene is also an anti-inflammatory. Natural anti-inflammatories are a vital part of disease prevention simply because strong circulation throughout the body is how organs are nourished and detoxed. Spirulina is also notably high in iron, calcium, zinc, potassium, magnesium, selenium, and phosphorus, all of which play a tremendous role in our overall health and longevity.

Chlorella shines in its ability to enhance detoxification. Of all algae, chlorella is at the very top of the totem pole in terms of chlorophyll content. Along with detoxification, the high chlorophyll content supports oxygenation of our blood and consequent energy production in all cells (O_2 = life-force). So, naturally, chlorella enhances physical stamina and energy. Studies have also proven chlorella reduces blood pressure and lowers cholesterol. Interestingly, the causes behind these benefits of chlorella have not yet been fully understood. Oh, the mysteries of nature!

I truly feel algae can play a significant role in our diet, and I'm confident the world will better understand why these foods are so important in the near future. Bottom line—gram for gram, algae have concentrations of nutrients unmatched by anything else. Naturally, all of the reasons above are part of why I am so partial to my Infinity formulas, of which algae are the biggest part.

I truly believe algae are literally the antidote for us overfed, yet undernourished, modern humans. Like we discussed in Chapter 1, it is worth noting that today, even unprocessed plant foods do not have the same nutrient content they did just a few decades ago because of the soil depletion from mass agriculture. However, this is not the case for algae! It's the same extraordinary nutrition that it was three and a half billion years ago.

I believe that before long, algae will be a much better understood and more utilized food on a global scale. As for how to introduce algae into your diet, start by adding it to your smoothies. Already, smoothies should have a role in your diet if they're made with genuinely healthy ingredients. And I'll share my favorite smoothie recipes in the back of this book.

It should be noted that in the 1970s, grass supplements like wheat grass and barley grass came about as a low-budget green food. The theory was "greens for pennies." But unfortunately the pretty price of grass supplements comes with drawbacks. Yes, grasses have *some* chlorophyll but nothing even close to that of algae. What many people are unaware of is that wheat grass (even juiced) is hard to digest and can be weakening for the gastrointestinal system. I say "pass" on these products. Algae and all other green foods are superior to wheat grass.

To sum it all up, introducing the right greens into your diet, ones that are high in chlorophyll and nutrients—whether kale, spinach, or algae—is about much more than just weight loss. You know, it's interesting how our modern diets focus so heavily on getting the "right" calories and nutrients. But think about it. Getting the calories and nutrients *in* is only half the picture. The other half is getting the toxic funk *out!* Removing the wear and tear from your internals makes it well worth the small effort of adding more chlorophyll-rich green foods to your diet. The main idea here is, we are honing a diet to enable our body to rejuvenate faster than it would break down. That's the ultimate key for longevity, life-force, and protection from disease.

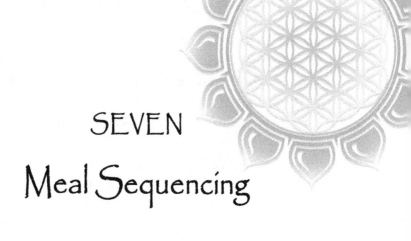

SEVEN

Meal Sequencing

Okay, here's the chapter you've been waiting for. We've learned a lot in the past six chapters about healthy eating and now it's time to apply what we've learned. Let's consider the sequencing of our meals and walk through a typical day, making certain that we're eating a healthy breakfast, a healthy lunch, and a healthy dinner.

Breakfast

Remember Mom repeating the old adage, *Breakfast is the most important meal of the day*? Well, we all know Mom was right. But Mom's advice needs just a little fine-tuning. Breakfast *is* important, but when, and what, you fuel your body with are what it really boils down to.

First, remember that when you wake up in the morning naturally your body is a little dehydrated. For me, when my feet hit the ground, it's at least eight ounces of pure water. No need to measure it though. Simply chug till your thirst is quenched. (More on water in the next chapter!) Shortly after that, I have a smoothie. This is the golden hour for adding nutrient-dense foods that provide vital nourishment for sustained energy, reflected in how you'll feel all day long.

First thing in the morning, your digestive system is just coming out of rest mode, making it important to start your day with easier-to-digest foods. That's why a smoothie is a brilliant option. It's liquid, drinkable nutrition. Like we talked about, make it a balanced meal by including easy to digest plant proteins, healthy raw fats, and natural complex carbohydrates from whole fruit. Remember my favorite smoothie is made with a banana, a round tablespoon of almond butter, purified water, and Infinity Greens. Now that's balance! It's satisfying, low-cal, nutrient rich, hydrating, and easy to digest. And you'll be impressed by how long this meal fuels the body. (More smoothie recipes to choose from in the Appendix!)

But wait—we seem to have skipped caffeine! Most of us start with coffee, after all. Starting with a nutritious breakfast reduces the need for as much caffeine. Nutrients are life force, allowing all the organs to function at their best. Drink a properly-made smoothie, and you'll find less of a need for those morning cups of joe.

If you really want caffeine, remember my preference is tea. Chai is my personal favorite. And we're not talking premade chai, already loaded with sugar, either. Simple black tea, brewed with ginger, cardamom, clove and nutmeg, is all it takes. Add a sprinkle of coconut sugar and a splash of milk if you wish. But have your smoothie first. Starting your day with caffeine first means a lot of stimulation right off the bat without healthy fuel to back it up. That often leads to undulating energy levels. And, if proper fuel isn't provided, the body compensates by lowering your metabolism. Among other effects on your health, this certainly doesn't help if weight loss is a concern.

A few hours after your smoothie is a great time to get more of those complex carbohydrates. Oatmeal is perfect, along with your natural sweetener of choice, like berries and a little honey. Add some healthy protein and fats with raw nuts and seeds or maybe a little yogurt. Eggs scrambled or fried in a little coconut oil (preferably in a cast iron pan) with sprouted grain bread or corn tortillas with beans can be a great option too.

The idea is to split your breakfast into smaller meals, allowing your digestive system some time in between the meals to do its work. We all know mornings can be hectic, trying to feed the dog, get the kids out the door, getting dressed and ready to take on the day, etc. Just another good reason to make a smoothie which really just takes a few minutes once it's a part of your routine. Later, when you're more settled into your day, take a break with oatmeal or eggs. This doesn't mean snacking and grazing all morning! We're talking well-defined meals.

What *not* to eat? We can start with the ever-popular processed cereals, even most of the "natural" ones. Read those ingredients: wheat flour, evaporated cane juice, safflower oil, and canola oil. And do I really need to get into pancakes and waffles swimming in high fructose corn syrup?

What about the eggs-bacon-potatoes combo? This seems to be the main menu item for breakfast in every diner in America. Well I say it's time to flip the script on this die-hard, outdated convention. Eggs are cool, but eating dense proteins (bacon, sausage, ham) combined with starchy foods (that heaping pile of hash browns) leads to that oh-so-sleepy feeling that should *not* be happening at the start of your day. Animal proteins and carbohydrates each require different kinds of enzymes supplied by your digestive system to break them down, meaning that your body has to work harder, thus draining you of energy. Save the food coma for Thanksgiving dinner and jumpstart your day with foods that will optimize your performance.

Lunch

Sure, breakfast is the most important meal because it sets the tone for your day. But don't stop there. As the day moves on, we want to continue the trend of making good decisions. Ever skip or work through lunch because you didn't have the time or because you had a big breakfast? Not ideal. Our ultimate goal is to maintain a *steady* stream of healthy energy and balanced blood sugar levels throughout the day. When you think blood sugar level, think energy level. We want to avoid becoming hypoglycemic (low blood sugar), with low energy—the outcome of going without fuel for more than four to five hours.

As with breakfast, eating smaller meals about every three to four hours is optimal in regulating those blood sugar levels. A larger meal for lunch means longer digestion time which comes with a drowsy, sluggish feeling in the middle of your afternoon. Eat a smaller lunch and then look forward to another healthy mini-meal later in the afternoon.

Lunchtime, since your digestive system has had time to rev up, is a good time for raw vegetables. Because of the rigidity of most vegetables, they're naturally harder to digest than something like a breakfast smoothie. So bring out the raw veggies at lunch and make yourself a tasty salad. And, no, not the chicken and iceberg lettuce one. What we want is a *real* salad. Mix it at home before you go to work. Remember to use those dark leafy greens. Throw in some sliced cucumber, celery, sauerkraut, carrots. Maybe some cherry tomatoes and a sprinkling of almonds or pumpkin seeds. Some sun-cured olives. Throw a tablespoon of ground flax seeds into the mix. Then top it with *real* salad dressing: the juice of a lemon, a tablespoon of olive oil, a little sea salt, a dash of cayenne pepper. It doesn't just have to be salads, either. Go with some complex carbs from grains like steamed quinoa or rice (brown or white is fine). Grains are good if you need to bulk up on calories. You'll find plenty of options in the Appendix.

Some people add fruit to their salad, liked sliced orange or strawberries. But there's one thing to keep in mind: combining fruit and vegetables tends to cause fermentation (yup, gas). So if you're eating fruits *and* vegetables, remember to eat your fruit first. Fruit digests in just a few minutes so you can have your salad shortly after.

Lunch Part II

In addition to your midday lunch—in keeping with the philosophy of maintaining your energy level—have a healthy mini-meal later in your workday. It'll act as a nice pick-me-up and is especially valuable in averting such disasters as what tends to occur about eight seconds after you get home from work. How many times, when you get home, have you headed straight for the pantry where you keep the chips and crackers?

Fruit can be perfect for your next meal after lunch. Natural sugars and fiber will iron out your blood sugar levels and help you maintain that steady energy. Remember that the simple-to-digest protein fats, like almond butter, can go well with fruit, like an apple, for more of a well-defined meal. Fruits mixed with raw nuts or seeds is a classic. Remember to "pass" on the roasted peanuts and cashews. Even better, have another smoothie! Or how about an Infinity Bar? Need I say I'm quite partial to my bars? A tasty, nutritious mini-meal is exactly why they were created.

Dinner

You've done well so far. Your breakfast and lunch have been comprised of nutritious, well-balanced, well-defined smaller meals. Now let's round out the day with a suitable dinner.

Dinner often tends to be an afterthought for people. It's the end of the day, we're tired, we're hungry, and, oh look, there's a drive-through! Don't mind if I do! Or, if we're able to bypass the drive-through, sometimes we fall victim to this popular end-of-the-day protocol: we come home and sit down to a gigantic meal of low quality animal protein and pasta, bread, or similar starchy foods—often revered as comfort foods. Of course there's nothing wrong with having these foods if the goal is to store fat on the backside. But since your dietary goals are likely a bit more enlightened, I bet you're willing to spend a little time thinking your dinner plans through.

So what's for dinner? Well, you just spent the day fueling your body with nutrition to propel you through the day's activities: work, working out, chasing the kids, pleasing the boss, dealing with customers—whatever your day demanded from you. So now, dinner is the time for nutrition that is *restorative*. And, naturally, as you'll recall from earlier in the book, a big part of this is protein. If you have meat in your diet, this is when to have it. Just remember, choosing premium proteins is critical for anyone who is serious about their health. Why not opt for the elite foods like fish? For the vegetarian options think lentils, tempeh, edamame, seeds, eggs, and rice and beans. Go a little lighter on the carbohydrates (fuel) at this time of day, especially those processed starchy ones. And remember to keep your fats healthy. Examples of healthy, delicious dinner meals? This is what the Appendix is for!

Don't forget that in the evening, when your body is less active, the food you stock up on is more apt to become stored as fat. This is part of why it's important that you eat at least a few hours before bedtime. That'll help your sleep pattern, too, which we'll cover in a little more detail later on.

But what about dessert or a snack for later at night? The late night sweet tooth is another one of those mysteries. Suddenly out of nowhere we might just crave some ice cream. Well, there are healthy ways to satisfy *that* desire. One of my personal evening favorites is whole yogurt with raw honey (*not* the low-fat sweetened yogurt!). It's a great pre-bedtime meal and just a small amount will do the trick. Interestingly, honey helps with the release of melatonin in the brain which is great for sleep.

Eating with the Seasons

It's worth noting that the foods you instinctively want to eat—your body's natural desires—change not just depending on the time of day, but also on the time of year. Generally, when temperatures are cooler, the body wants cooked foods which are, by nature, warming to the body. Conversely, in warmer climates, we naturally gravitate towards foods like raw fruits and vegetables which are inherently cooling for the body. In other words, your cravings in the middle of a winter in North Dakota will be much different than what your body craves in the middle of summer in Arizona. This phenomenon, though well-known and well-defined in Chinese medicine, is given much less attention here in the West than I think it deserves.

Listen to your body when you're planning your meals. But strive for a healthy balance. In general, most people need to add more raw fruits and vegetables into their diet for at least most of the year. But take advantage of your body's extra need for them during the warmer season. Since raw plant foods are high in water-content and enzymes, this makes them cleansing, especially for the gastrointestinal tract. That's always a good thing but especially in the summer.

If it's the winter and you're eating more cooked foods, make sure they're the right cooked foods. One thing to remember is that certain nutrients are lost in the heating-cooking process that could be especially beneficial in cold weather, like immune-boosting vitamin C. But some nutrients, particularly minerals, are heat stable and can actually become more absorbable after cooking.

On the subject of cooked food, I am often asked if there really is any potential harm with using microwaves. I'll explain this in simple terms. Microwaves work by penetrating food with radiation creating intermolecular friction via vibrating molecules. This friction is what heats the food. Research has thoroughly proven that the molecular structures within microwaved food partially break down producing a compound called nitric oxide. The biochemical reaction nitric oxide propagates in the body is the formation of free radicals, which then produce inflammation. Inflammation in the body has the potential to weaken everything. (We will talk more about free radicals and inflammation in Chapter 13.) I understand it's hard to believe that something so mainstream as a microwave could actually be harmful. But consider it's only one example among many. Are sugar and fried food not similar examples? They all fit within the modern theme, "if it's tasty, cheap and easy then it's a go", – all put upon the masses with the most impressive marketing. I wouldn't say microwaved food on occasion would necessarily do harm. But it's not something to do on a lifestyle basis either. So I say take a 'pass' on the microwave and use your convection oven (a superior upgrade) instead. Any way that we can minimize exposure to free radicals from something so basic as a microwave is worth the minimal compromise of convenience.

Now back to the question of cooked versus raw – how do you make sure you've got the right balance? Well, as you know by now, I believe that we have an instinctive sense of what's best for us. Listen to your body's wisdom—something you will become better at over time. And look for clues your body is giving you. If you're often cold, then you likely need more cooked foods that have a warming effect on the body. Naturally, the opposite is true if you're often hot. More raw foods would be the answer.

Congratulations! You've eaten healthy all day. Breakfast, lunch, dinner. When it comes to the quality and content of your meals, you have to think of your body like it's a car. Pumping whatever you want into the gas tank won't necessarily get you very far. Sure, it might drive, but will it drive well? And for how long? And what will be the long-term effects? We're often smart about what gas or oil goes into our cars. Shouldn't we be just as smart with our bodies? Or even smarter?

When we fuel our bodies with quality nutrition, we have more energy, we think more clearly, we don't have those cravings for foods that aren't beneficial for us, we become more resistant to disease, and, all in all, we just *feel* better, making the great benefit worth the little effort and discipline it requires.

EIGHT

Digestive Health

Here's a big-picture consideration for you: everything we've discussed so far with respect to your diet greatly affects your *digestive health*, a vital pillar of your well-being. Your digestive system plays two critical roles: it extracts nutrition from the foods you eat and it eliminates toxins from the body. When the digestive system is strong, it does an outstanding job in both roles. When it's compromised by poor diet, it does a poor job. Your diet, indeed your lifestyle, amplifies, for good or for bad, your digestive system's performance.

In fact, because of the dual-role nature of the digestive system, a poor diet actually *compounds* the problem of poor nutrition. You're not taking in quality nutritive foods in the first place, and the nutrients you *are* taking in aren't being properly extracted for the body's use because of the weakened digestive system. It's an unhealthy spiral.

The good news is digestive health isn't very complicated. It all comes down to what we've learned thus far. For optimal health, your body needs more plant foods—fruits and vegetables, along with unprocessed whole grains and healthy fats. Additionally, it requires some elimination—like cutting out processed sugar, flour, and cheap animal protein. Without fiber from plant foods, everything slows down. We've talked about how weakening flour can be, a significant fiber-less ingredient in so many diets. Rumor has it that the average American gets half of his or her calories from flour and sugar! Scary, isn't it? Animal protein, as mentioned above, another major ingredient in the typical diet, doesn't do your digestive system any favors either. If meat and/or dairy are regular parts of your diet, take breaks from them every now and then. Give your digestive system a chance to recuperate and strengthen itself. That said, there are a few more details about diet and the digestive system that you should become familiar with.

What and How You Eat

It's probably not surprising that some of the best foods for your gastrointestinal system are foods that are easy to digest. The hard-to-digest foods we've identified (especially animal protein and flour) can have a tendency to accumulate in the gastrointestinal tract, slowing things down, allowing toxins more opportunity to be absorbed through the intestines back into the body. This also interferes with the body's ability to soak up beneficial nutrients.

What *may* be surprising, however, is that some raw vegetables aren't always easy to digest either. While raw veggies aren't foods that accumulate in the gastrointestinal system, they *can* make it work hard. Remember in Chapter 6 we talked about the presence of cellulose in the coarser, more rigid vegetables (like kale, chard, collard greens, and broccoli), that makes them harder to digest when raw versus when cooked. Strike a balance by mixing it up. Also remember my philosophy about tossing these greens into the blender! Raw, easy to digest, and chlorophyll—score! Give my kale sauce a try! It's a favorite of many. (See the Appendix.)

Cooked or not, it's important to chew your food thoroughly. Ever notice how fast many people eat these days? Much of the world is in a hurry. But chewing is Phase One of digestion, and it's super important. There are digestive enzymes in your saliva that begin breaking down food before it's even swallowed. Take your time when you eat. You'll get more taste out of your food and you'll make things a lot easier on your digestive system.

Your Internal Chemistry

One especially unappealing consequence of a poor diet is internal parasites. These are more common than we like to believe. We all have them, to some degree. The most common is a yeast fungus called candida which thrives on processed sugar and flour. Alcohol, too. Candida weakens the walls of the intestines, often creating food sensitivities. Along with removing the foods that candida thrives on, I recommend doing battle against candida from time to time with foods and herbs that are known to kill it. Raw garlic is a classic one. To be effective however, it has to be truly raw, unheated garlic. Chewing raw garlic can be a painful for the tongue (not to mention can have socially unfashionable effects). Dicing it up very finely to be washed down with a glass of water will spare you from having to chew it. Parasites hate raw garlic. And there's a whole host of similar parasite fighting superfoods and herbs that can be found in the supplement section of any store. Do your research to find what antiparasitics are best for you. The good news is, once strong and balanced, your digestive system can keep candida and other parasites at bay. Remember that a digestive system in a weakened state leads to an unhealthy internal chemistry which, in turn, weakens the whole body. It weakens your very life force. And consider this – the digestive tract is where the majority of serotonin is created in the body. Serotonin is what has a direct impact on our mood. That alone is reason enough to maintain a healthy digestive system. It's worth stating again: digestive health is a pillar of *overall* health.

Poor diets cause poor internal chemistry because of the lack of nutrition (obviously), but also because of the typical components of the common diet; namely, sugar, flour, and lack of fiber. Fiber, of course, helps move things along in your system, thus making it

61

more difficult for parasites, or any toxic material for that matter, to stick around. There are two kinds of fiber: soluble and insoluble. Soluble (typically from plant foods) breaks down, dissolving in your system. Insoluble (typically from grains), doesn't digest. (One exception is oats, which are a great soluble fiber.) Insoluble fiber still plays an important role, though, because it adds bulk to your food, helping satisfy your appetite with fewer calories. But ironically, too much insoluble fiber can be constipating. Soluble fiber plays the more important role, keeping things moving through the gastrointestinal tract.

As I mentioned in Chapter 2, flax and chia seeds are an amazing source of soluble fiber, superior alternatives to other fiber supplements like psyllium husk. Both of these seeds lubricate the gastrointestinal system perfectly. Either grind them up in a blender or soak them in water for maximum effect. I often mix a round tablespoon of ground flax seeds into a salad. Sprouted, raw flaxseed crackers are a great product, but the less adulterated products are always better. Also, try soaking your other nuts and seeds in water overnight. When nuts, like almonds for example, are soaked they actually release natural preservatives. These preservatives are what protect nuts in nature, giving them a chance to sprout and grow before they are broken down by bacteria and insects. This is why soaking nuts and seeds will make a big difference in the digestibility. Or shop for nuts and seeds that have already been soaked and dehydrated, commonly referred to as "sprouted." This adds a nice crispness that makes them a really delicious food.

Cleaning the System

Speaking of taking breaks from poor nutritional habits, many people do cleanses from time to time. Some people will fast for days and even longer as a way to detox, although some do it for spiritual reasons, too. The idea is to cleanse the body of toxins that have built up, especially in the colon. I wouldn't necessarily advocate a heroic detoxifying cleanse for everyone, but I wouldn't stop you, either. It's fascinating how the body will truly cleanse itself if it's allowed the chance to do so.

One way to do a cleanse is by utilizing a liquid diet exclusively. Juicing fresh fruit and veggies (not pre-bottled products) can be good for such a cleanse, but I'm a bigger fan of smoothies, the advantage being that you're getting the whole food including the cleansing soluble fiber that comes with it. It's true that juicing gives the digestive system a break while still providing the nutrients, but so does blended food, especially if you're using a high-power blender which really breaks things down. A quality blender can be money well spent.

Many people will undergo periodic colon irrigation, administered by colonic hygienists. An enema is a lighter-version colonic that can be self-administered. Another option for flushing the system out, top to bottom, is a non-invasive technique called Shatkarma that goes all the way back to the ancient health practices of Ayurveda. Essentially, this entails drinking a liter of salt water that you can mix yourself with non-iodized sea salt and purified water to make it comparable to ocean water. This is an extremely effective cleanse. The body can't absorb salt water, so it travels through the intestines, top to bottom. Just make sure you have a bathroom handy for the next couple hours as you'll have at least a few substantial bowel movements. This is something that I did for years, and I think it's great. (Note: this is the only reason you would ever drink salt water since salt water is dehydrating, but there's no harm in drinking a liter for the sake of bowel cleansing.) Search online for the how-to's. It's a well-known practice.

For a digestive system that's slow to the point of constipation, you might be thinking about laxatives. I don't recommend using them except for rare occasions since, over time, your system can become dependent on them. If and when you really need it, I'd suggest senna, which is a natural (herbal) laxative. Aloe latex is a stronger natural option.

Fasts, colonics, Shatkarma flushes—these can all be effective. But more to the point, I'd simply recommend a diet that is cleansing in general. Even just a few days after removing meat, too many dairy products, sugar, and foods with flour, you'll likely be able to sense toxic funk leaving your body. Not to say that it's necessarily going to feel good. For a few days you may feel a sensation of a hangover since an increased volume of toxins is moving through the bloodstream to be excreted through the gastro-system. Chlorophyll from green food, nature's purifier of blood, is an important ally here. After a cleanse such as this, you might just decide to leave the less-than-healthy things out of your diet all the time, naturally gravitating towards the healthy—cleansing—foods.

Strengthening Your System

Besides a cleansing diet, a major way to strengthen your internal chemistry is with healthy bacteria. *Unhealthy* intestinal bacteria have become a common theme with the prevalence of modern junk foods. The *right* kind of bacteria supports digestion among other things in the body. When healthy bacteria settle in, they also become defenders, greatly enhancing your immune system. We can get healthy bacteria in raw, fermented foods like sauerkraut. A source becoming very popular these days is kombucha tea, a fizzy, fermented beverage. It's a tasty drink that's actually been around since ancient times. Probiotic supplements can play a major role, too. These include bacterial blends of acidophilus, bifidus, and lactobacillus. Before the days of probiotic supplements we got our healthy intestinal bacteria from the dirt caked on raw veggies coming from right out of the garden. This is still possible if you have your own garden but not from the produce at your local store since the probiotic-rich dirt has already been rinsed off.

The microorganisms that inhabit your digestive tract—your intestinal flora—heavily influence your digestive health. How do you know if your intestinal flora is healthy? The most accurate gauge is your bowel movements. Fiber, coupled with a predominance of healthy bacteria, give bulk. A healthy bowel movement is sizable and, well, there's just no other way to say it, satisfying.

And while we're on the subject of bowel movements, you should be having at least one a day. Regular bowel movements are important for making sure that toxins don't linger in the intestines too long for the reasons I mentioned. A good diet aids this regularity. For enhanced gastro-mobility, keep in mind that effective and common intestinal lubricants include coconut oil, flaxseeds, chia seeds, papaya, and prunes. And here's a little-known cause of constipation: our Western-designed toilets. They're too tall! Sitting up high shortens the colon into a position that is less than ideal for things to move along. Bringing your feet up, even just a few inches, puts your body in more of a squat position which solves this problem. Get creative and put something under your feet, making way for things to more easily travel their course. It will make a difference.

Other ways to strengthen your digestive system include enzymes, which are important for breaking foods down for proper digestion. Where do you find these? Raw fruits and veggies. Enzyme supplements can be useful but aren't for everyone due to their blood thinning effect. Ginger is also helpful for digestion by ramping the up the spleen which strengthens your digestive fire.

Other Factors

Naturally, water also plays a role in digestive health. We'll talk in the next chapter about hydration. For now, suffice it to say that many of us are walking around slightly dehydrated most of the time. It's no coincidence that many of us are also walking around slightly constipated most of the time, too. Drink water! Ideally, do the majority of hydrating through the day and less with meals. Hydrating during meals does slightly dilute your digestive enzymes. At the very least, try to avoid cold drinks with food. While cold drinks during mealtime is a common theme, they do in fact dampen your digestion.

Exercise is another factor. Regular exercise keeps thing moving, helping you stay regular. It also helps build your core strength which is important in maintaining your internal structure. One of the lesser-known consequences of obesity is that the internal organs have a tendency to not sit quite right, often getting squeezed and scrunched by the fat that's built up around them. There's simply less room in the gut resulting in a slowing-down of the food moving through the intestines.

Oral Health

Did you know your digestive health can be reflected in your breath? While the majority of toxins that enter our bodies are excreted by the digestive system, some are eliminated via exhalation. When you stop and think about it, the mouth is a part of the digestive system! Bad breath can be a symptom of poor digestive health, reflecting an unhealthy internal chemistry.

You don't need me to tell you to brush your teeth. But here's something you might want to think about: toxins that are eliminated by exhalation have a tendency to congregate on your tongue, mostly on the back of the tongue where it goes unnoticed. That's right. Metabolic waste and unhealthy bacteria get stuck there. This accumulation normally presents itself as a mild white film. In front of a mirror stick your tongue out as far as you can. Do you see it? Yup, it's toxins accumulating on your tongue—yuck! This creates two problems. It causes bad breath, and it allows the toxins to re-circulate through the body as you end up swallowing them back down as the food you eat scrapes it off as you swallow.

Though this may sound like a minor issue, it really is deserving of our attention. A small amount of toxins may not sound like a big deal, but a lifetime of small amounts of toxins being re-circulated through the body every day will definitely add up, potentially to be reflected somewhere down the road. Fortunately, there's an easy fix. A simple tongue brush/scraper. I recommend the GUM brand. One side is a brush specially designed to brush the tongue and the other side is a scraper for scraping off the stuff you've brushed loose. A regular toothbrush won't do it. The bristles of a tongue brush are much coarser. Thirty seconds a day is all it takes, preferably first thing in the morning since the toxins and bacteria build up mostly overnight. Do it, and it'll help maintain a healthy internal chemistry, as well as clean breath.

Bad breath is one of those taboo subjects. Nobody will tell you when you have it. After scraping your tongue, smell your tongue brush and tell me you're not surprised. Using a tongue brush might be new to you and so it might require some practice to get the hang of it. Like I mentioned, the majority of the toxic material is toward the back of the tongue where it's hard to see, and reach. Getting back there with your brush may not be the most pleasant sensation at first, but it's something you'll quickly get used to. Take it slow. There's no need to make yourself gag or brush so hard that your tongue bleeds.

The tongue scraper on the other side of the brush is equally important to scrape off the funk that has been loosened by brushing. Tongue scrapers are available without the brush on the other side, but the brush and scraper together are far more effective. Do this daily, and soon enough you'll get used to it to the point where your mouth won't feel quite right if you skip it. The rare occasion I don't brush my tongue I notice a slightly unpleasant taste all day. After you've experienced this contrast yourself, I promise you'll wonder how we all didn't catch on to this sooner! And, by the way, what it might just do for your love-life could be awesome. Please take my advice and brush your tongue.

A note about mouthwash. The irony is hilarious. The alcohol in mouthwash actually wipes out the healthy bacteria in your mouth, essentially making way for the unhealthy bacteria to dominate the scene. At best, mouthwash temporarily covers up the smell, only so that it can come back later with a vengeance. Breath mints and gum are similar disasters. Unhealthy bacteria thrive on sugar, as well as the xylitol in sugar-free gum. It's hard not to feel sorry for the many people walking around chewing gum cheerily thinking their breath smells better when in fact they're making it worse.

The importance of a healthy gastrointestinal system cannot be emphasized enough. It's a pillar of your health and an accurate indicator of it, too. But proper digestive health doesn't require rocket science. Eat the right foods at the right times. Cut out sugar, flour, cheap animal protein, low-grade oils, and slow-to-digest foods. Get plenty of soluble fiber. And that's all there is to it. Simple. The best part? Within no time, you'll find that your digestive system is getting stronger, and reflected by everything else in your body getting stronger, too. Give the protocols we've covered a "go" for one month and I can assure that you'll find the impact anything but subtle.

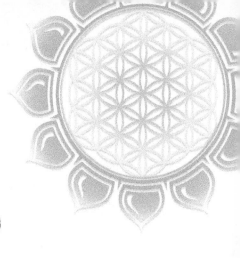

NINE
H_2O

This is an easy one to take for granted which is why it never seems to get the attention it deserves. But without it, we sure wouldn't last very long. It's one of the pillars of life. Of course I'm talking about water. And because it's what we put the most of into our bodies, it warrants some serious consideration. After all, our bodies are seventy-percent water! Water that is clean and pure is vital for so many things, some of the most notable being the proper functioning of our organs, a strong immune system, maintaining energy and vitality, mental clarity, and longevity. Thankfully, getting this right isn't hard! But there are a few key factors.

The Problem with Water Today

Unfortunately, pure water is not all that easy to come by. Most water available today (tap and bottled) is far from pure and is not the same water we were drinking a hundred years ago (or even ten years ago, for that matter). Much of it is contaminated with chlorine, fluoride, lead, mercury, pesticides, and bacteria (to mention just a few). In urbanized areas where recycled water is used, testing reveals even trace amounts of pharmaceuticals due to them passing through the user's body. Yikes! Impure water might well be why we get sick more than we think we should, or develop allergies due to a weak immune system, or often feel just okay instead of energized and really alive.

So where can you find the cleanest, purest water? It may be no surprise that it turns out that *fresh spring water*, assuming it's free of contaminants, is the best water. Well water is a close second to fresh spring water, again purity being the determining factor.

Filtering is a Start

The problem, however, is that we don't all have access to a fresh, pure spring or a well. So what to do? Well, an inexpensive first step would be a filter. A simple carbon filtration system will remove large sediment and chlorine. These carbon filters are the filters that attach to your faucet or come inside the common pitchers. You might want to consider a carbon filter even if you have well water. Well water can sometimes be a little over-mineralized, creating a kind of metallic taste. A carbon filter should take care of that.

You can go a step further and get a whole house carbon filtration system where all of your water is filtered before it runs through any of the faucets in your home. Any plumber can install one for you.

However, where recycled water is used in more populated areas, carbon filtration is definitely not adequate for the healthy lifestyle we're going for. Sure these systems can take out sediment and chlorine (chlorine is a large molecule which a carbon filter has no problem trapping), but they are inadequate for filtering out most of the other contaminants. This is very important. The filtration of both pitchers and refrigerators is nowhere close to sufficient. The only ways to thoroughly filter your water are with a reverse-osmosis filter or a distiller.

A reverse-osmosis filter works by squeezing the water through a pressurized filter membrane. The pores in the membrane are the size of a water molecule, allowing virtually only pure water molecules to pass through. The filters typically need to be changed once a year; otherwise, the system doesn't really require any maintenance. These, too, are units that any plumber can install for you under your kitchen sink, and they're generally no more than a few hundred bucks. Still, if you're not sure about spending the money on a reverse-osmosis filter, try renting one first. That way, you have nothing to lose. Plus, maintenance is typically included.

The distiller option works by having the water steamed and then pressed through a filter. These are more expensive than reverse-osmosis systems, but the filtration is a little better, too. Both reverse-osmosis systems and distillation filters are generally installed under the kitchen sink with a separate faucet on the countertop. At a minimum, I believe a good quality reverse-osmosis system should be considered a basic household amenity.

Mineralizing and Ionizing

Reverse-osmosis systems and water distillation systems do present one minor issue. The filtering process, being as thorough as it is, filters out trace minerals. Trace minerals include over seventy minerals that are found in spring water. What's the role of these trace minerals? They make the water more absorbable, and they're beneficial for the body on their own account, too. There are trace mineral products available at most natural food stores for adding to your water after filtration. Of course you can get these minerals in food, as well.

There's another thing that sets spring water apart: ionization. In springs or streams or rivers, water rushing and churning over rocks creates a bonding of water molecules into hexagonal structures (this is why snowflakes are hexagonal shaped). This helps explain the surface tension of water—the way water holds itself together. Think of how you can fill a glass slightly higher than the top of the glass without the water spilling over. It's this ionization that makes it more absorbable by the body. With municipal water, you actually have to drink more of it to quench your body's thirst, since much of it passes right through!

If money's not a factor, there are such things as water ionizers. These are units that sit on your countertop. They filter the water and add minerals and use electricity to create an ionization comparable to the churning of flowing spring water, creating the bonding of water molecules. The drawback, besides cost, is that water ionizers only use carbon filters, so you'll still need a reverse-osmosis filter or distiller for the water to pass through first, for the purpose of getting the water free of small contaminants. If money *is* a factor, don't sweat it. I do feel these products are a little over-hyped. The notion that people feel better using them is likely because they are simply drinking more water since the ionizers do improve the taste with minerals. And you can alkalize your body with a healthy diet anyway. The most important thing here is water purity. And of course drinking enough of it.

Bottled Water

What about bottled water? Can you really get the purity that the bottling companies advertise? Well, maybe. Most bottled water is reverse-osmosis filtered. Some companies advertise natural spring water, which should theoretically provide the minerals, but it's worth noting that the water ions begin to dissipate after sitting for about a month. The more critical factor is the purity of the spring which, to the consumer, is really unknown.

Then there's the bottling itself: plastic versus glass. Plastic is made of petroleum which inevitably leaches its own contaminants, especially if the water's been sitting in the bottle for months (and invariably it has). If you're out somewhere and you're dehydrated and you grab a plastic bottle of water, no big deal. But for your everyday drinking water, opt for water sold in glass. And if you're on the go throughout your day, then take water with you in a glass or steel bottle rather than plastic. If you're using a delivery service that provides spring water to your home in five-gallon containers, I suggest a service that will provide glass containers instead of plastic. Just be careful muscling around what adds up to about fifty pounds of water and glass! (Tip: wrap a slightly damp towel around the glass container first. Then pick it up with a bear hug. You'll get a better grip.)

Whatever you do, find a way—within your budget—to do *something*. Keep in mind that not all municipal water is bad. If you live in certain rural areas, for instance, your local water may, in fact, be sourced from a spring or a well. But if not, at the very least, filter your water with a good reverse-osmosis system. The common pitcher with a carbon filter is simply inadequate.

Some Notes on Hydration

Okay, so now we know the importance of pure water. Make sure you're getting the best available. And plenty of it. How much water should you be drinking? Listen to your body. Most people are consistently in a state of mild dehydration without even being aware of it. It's kind of the norm. And when you think about it, this just might be a function of our inferior tap water. The most common water often doesn't taste that good. So we don't go out of our way to drink it. It's instinctual—the body doesn't want it the same way it wants pure water.

If you find yourself craving cold ice water, it's likely an indication you're dehydrated. Dehydration produces a slightly higher body temperature and the body wants to cool down, hence the craving for something cold. If your urine is consistently a darker yellow color, that's another sign that you're not getting enough water. Migraines are often caused by dehydration, too. And daytime sluggishness generally comes with it. The body is wrapped in a thin layer of facia that aids in your body parts moving smoothly. When dehydrated, cells in the facia shrink, and things don't move as well, often giving the body a chronic mild ache. Also the body's ability to remove toxic waste from cells becomes stagnant which is reflected by everything slowing down and becoming weaker. As always, pay attention to what your body is telling you. *Everything* works better when you're properly hydrated.

Ironically, a lot of dehydration is caused by things that we're drinking. Coffee is dehydrating. So is alcohol. Even sports drinks can be because they're full of sugar. After all, what does it take for your body to detoxify all that sugar? Water! (Water is the universal solvent for any toxin in the body.) Sports drinks are overhyped, false-advertised products. Quench your thirst with what's worked best ever since humans began to populate the earth: water. Make the majority of your hydration with unadulterated pure H_2O!

A side note about when to drink the majority of your water: as I mentioned in Chapter 7, it's important to drink one to two cups of pure water when your feet hit the floor first thing in the morning. Naturally, the body is in a state of mild dehydration after a night's sleep. Tea and coffee are acceptable to have *after* your water. And then of course the idea is to stay hydrated through-out the day. Because of the variables of body type, body size, and climate, it's hard to put a number on exactly how much water to drink. A general rule is one to two liters per day. Naturally if you're hiking all day in a dry climate you're going to drink more. Whilst drinking water that's adequately pure, trust your body's instincts and continue to satisfy your thirst exclusively with water rather than bottled drinks. A helpful gauge is the color of your urine. Light yellow is what we're shooting for.

You know what's also good at helping you to stay hydrated? High-water content foods. Just another reason to consume fresh fruits and vegetables. Grapes, apples, pears, berries, cucumbers, watermelon, and celery are just a few of the excellent sources of hydrating foods. Now that's pure water!

A note about hydrating during meals: it's less than ideal for the majority of hydrating to be *with* your meals which has inter-estingly become the norm. The key is to keep yourself hydrated throughout the day rather than hydrating when you sit down to eat. As we mentioned in the digestion chapter, water will dilute, however slightly, your digestive enzymes. Try to leave a window of thirty minutes before and after your meals to curb your water intake. If you're hydrating properly all day, that shouldn't be a problem. Try it. You'll find this becomes the body's natural preference. Of course if you're thirsty when you sit down to eat, then drink up. Hydration is a bigger priority than enzymes.

A note about the water from your shower: when unfiltered hot (municipal tap) water is sprayed from a faucet, the chlorine instantly turns to gas which is then inhaled. More chlorine can be absorbed by the body during a ten minute shower than by drinking chlorinated water all day! Filtering your drinking water is vital, but don't forget to filter your bathing water. A simple, inexpensive (less than thirty bucks) carbon filter from your local home improvement store can solve this problem for you. The shower head screws off, the filter screws onto the pipe, and then the shower head screws onto the filter. Easy. The whole-house water conditioner mentioned above also takes care of the chlorine for your showers, and all of your other faucets as well.

Okay, this all might seem like a lot of information for something as basic as water. But it's vitally important to give your body the best water possible, and taking a few easy steps towards making this happen has definite rewards. Plus, it gives you just that much less to worry about. Bottom line: being well hydrated with pure water makes everything in your body work far better. So drink up!

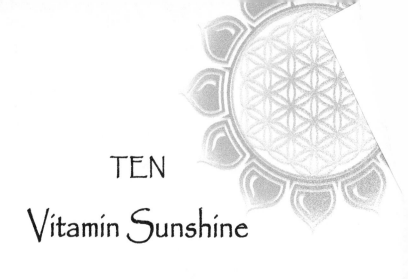

TEN

Vitamin Sunshine

Like we've talked about with food and water, we could all stand to get just a little more back to the basics. The elements we can get directly from Mother Nature rarely need a lot of modification. Here's another one: sunshine!

The Importance of Vitamin D

As you may know, vitamin D deficiency has become a serious health issue here in the Western world. And why is vitamin D so import-ant? For a whole host of reasons! For starters, its deficiency can be linked to today's prevalence of osteoporosis. Vitamin D metabolizes with calcium in the body helping to maintain sturdy bones. It's also a vital part of the immune system: one of the lesser-known but critical attributes of vitamin D is that it provides essential support in helping the body to remove toxins from your cells, effectively enhancing the life cycles of them, strengthening your body's defenses against autoimmune diseases and even cancer.

Now here's the issue: sunshine is, by far, the most generous source of vitamin D available. However, in an attempt to avoid skin damage and cancer, we slather sunscreen (containing toxic chemi-cals that are absorbed through the skin and enter the bloodstream) all over our bodies which ultimately ends up preventing the intake of vitamin D! During my lectures about vitamin D deficiency being linked to the overuse of sunscreen, I would get some blank stares. We have been thoroughly convinced via effective product marketing that we are doing something good for ourselves by wearing sunscreen any and every time we are in the sun. Reality check— there's a spell to be broken here. Living vitamin D deficient is a bigger deal than most people realize. And it gets even worse. To make up for our lack of vitamin D from the sun, we take potentially toxic vitamin D that is extracted from lambskin. Something is definitely wrong with this picture.

Moderation and the Right Protection

The keys are moderating your time under the sun as well as the timing of your exposure to it. Indeed, it is *very* important to prevent over-exposure to the sun which can otherwise cause free-radical damage. However, eliminating a vital element we receive from the sun on a regular basis is not a good solution either.

The target scenario is a short time in the sunshine with broad skin exposure. To get your vitamin D, five to ten minutes in the middle of the day in shorts and a tank top is likely adequate for fair-skinned people. Or up to twenty minutes if you're darker-skinned. Over time, tannins build in the skin which is the body's natural sun protection.

Now, the time of day that we're getting our sun exposure is very important. Sunshine comes to us in both UVA and UVB rays. It's the UVA radiation that causes potential damage to the skin. And it's the UVB radiation where we get our vitamin D. In the middle of the day when the sun is highest in the sky, UVB rays are plentiful. But when it's lower on the horizon, in the morning and evening hours, when the rays come through the atmosphere at an angle, the atmosphere filters out most of the vitamin D-forming UVB rays.

For that short period in the middle of the day, it's important to take advantage of direct, unscreened, unadulterated, pure sunshine. Let the sun's rays do their job, forming vitamin D on the surface of the skin which will then be absorbed into the bloodstream. Important side note: vitamin D is formed both within the skin cells as well as in the oils on the surface of the skin. It can take up to two days for vitamin D in the oils on the skin to be absorbed into the body. So for vitamin D's sake, avoid using soap on the arms and legs (assuming your arms and legs are what you primarily have exposed to the sun) which can literally wash the vitamin D away. Rinsing is okay. Use soap where you need it (armpits, privates, etc.). Don't worry—you're not going to stink if you don't use it on your arms and legs! By the way, younger people produce more vitamin D on their skin than older people, one reason that osteoporosis generally shows up later in life. Older or younger, the key is both timing and maximum surface area of skin exposed to the sun. Hence, my suggestion of shorts and a tank top. Or why not a little topless sunbathing in the backyard? The benefit is very real making it unquestionably worth the small amount of time and effort it takes.

Ah, but what if you're planning an activity that's going to involve being out in the sun all day? On the beach, maybe, or out on a boat? Sunscreens are necessary then, aren't they? Maybe, but first, there are better options than chemically made sunscreens. By the way, know what's in chemically made sunscreens? How's this for an ingredient list: oxybenzone, avobenzone, octisalate, octocrylene, homosalate, and octinoxate. What?? These chemicals have been linked to skin allergies and hormone imbalances. Yup. They're toxins that seep into the skin and accumulate in the body. No thanks. Go mineral rather than chemical. Use zinc oxide sunscreens. This is the sunscreen that may go on leaving your skin a bit white. But it's more natural, safer, and very effective. (I've actually found some brands that don't turn your skin white. You'll just have to try them.)

Incidentally, did you know that when manufacturers of sunscreens rate their product by SPF (Sunscreen Protection Factor), they're assuming you're rubbing one ounce of sunscreen on the body. That's one shot glass. Outside of the laboratory, nobody is putting on the amount of sunscreen necessary to reach the advertised SPF. A sunscreen with an SPF of 30 (meaning it theoretically provides 30 times the protection that bare skin provides) might, in reality, only be about a 10 given the amount most people use. Really your best sunscreen is shade, like a beach umbrella or a straw hat that shades your face and neck. When you're at the beach and you want to take a dip in the water, jump in, get your sun exposure, then jump out and hit the shade again. But if shade is *not* an option, then yes, use sunscreen.

If you spend a lot of your time out in the sun on a regular basis, it may be worth considering investing in some SPF clothing, kind of a new thing. The average cotton t-shirt has an SPF factor between only 5 and 10. Fine if you're not out in the sun all day. But if you're constantly exposed to long days in the sun on a regular basis, it may be worth checking out the lines of "sun protection" clothing on the market these days, generally made from cotton woven with zinc. This clothing can provide all the SPF you would ever need.

There is one more important factor with sun protection. Diet affects your body's natural sun protection! Like with every organ and function of the body, our diet makes everything weaker or stronger—the skin included. The quality of fats in your diet is the big one. In particular, the common omega-6 oils are a weak material for building skin and collagen and can essentially make the skin more vulnerable to sun damage. These are the oils rampant in the category of packaged foods—yet another important reason to be an ingredients reader.

A Note about Skin Care

While we're on the subject, this is a good time to talk about skin care in general. Most people don't realize that the chemical sunscreen ingredients listed above are in a lot of everyday skin care products. You may be using sunscreen without even knowing it! Skin is the body's largest organ and deserves to be free of toxic chemicals. Always be aware of what you're putting on your skin. It's a sensitive and a semi-permeable membrane, meaning that stuff can get both in and out. Did you know that antiperspirant deodorants contain aluminum? It's time to consider that the use of heavy metals for the purpose of clogging pores just might not be the most intelligent course of action. The idea should be to stay away from using *anything* that clogs the pores; after all, many toxins are eliminated through the pores!

For any skin care products you use, stick with the natural options. Want a good anti-aging moisturizer? Try olive oil, high in vitamin E and a superior upgrade from any lotion. The key is the way in which you apply it. In the shower, rub about a tablespoon of olive oil onto your body, head to toe. Rinse for another minute, and then towel dry. Your skin won't feel oily if done this way. And olive oil does not block pores.

Clothe your skin with natural materials. Wear cotton, cashmere, wool, hemp, or linen (most rayon is okay). Stay away from clothes made from petroleum like polyester which constantly gives off toxic gas. Rid your closet of acrylics, acetates, and nylons (except for your disco onesie and Halloween costume, of course). And use natural detergents. The idea is to remove pollutants from our everyday lifestyle. All of these factors add up over time. The skin gets replaced every twenty-eight days so, like many lifestyle changes, you'll notice a difference after just a month of taking better care of your skin.

Other Sources of Vitamin D

Back to vitamin D! Depending on where you are, in the winter months, it's often not as easy to get the vitamin D you need from the sun. Even on a sunny day, the sun is going to be lower in the sky, comparable to where it is in the mornings and evenings during the summer. Don't despair. Vitamin D is fat soluble, meaning that it can be stored for months in your fat cells. Plus, there are other ways to get vitamin D. Eggs and salmon are decent sources of vitamin D. But note that farm-raised salmon has only about a fourth of the vitamin D that wild-caught has. Wild-picked mushrooms have a respectable amount of vitamin D too. Interestingly, vitamin D forms on the surface of the mushroom from UVB radiation. Store-bought mushrooms don't have vitamin D since they are grown indoors. However, if you set your newly purchased mushrooms out in the sun, they will, in fact, produce vitamin D. Adequate data as to how much vitamin D this really provides is lacking, but any amount of vitamin D is valuable.

Winter, by the way, reveals another important attribute of the sun's rays. When the eyes interact with sunshine, the body produces serotonin, improving mood. Yup, the "winter blues" is a real thing. But you can get the winter blues at any time of year if you're indoors all the time and your eyes are not exposed to sunshine. The rays of the sun necessary to produce serotonin don't pass through glass. So even sitting next to a sunny window won't help. Plastic, however, like in most sunglasses, is conducive for the rays necessary for the production of serotonin.

To compensate for whatever UVB radiation you may not be getting in the winter, I don't recommend resorting to vitamin-D supplements. As I mentioned, vitamin D3 supplements are made from a waxy substance called lanolin that's taken from lamb-skin. Doesn't sound like anything I'm very keen on ingesting, how about you? And as with other supplements, it's actually easy to take too much vitamin D. An excess of manufactured vitamin D in the bloodstream has proven to be harmful for the kidneys. You don't have to worry about vitamin D toxicity if you're getting your vitamin D naturally—from the sun or from foods. Overdosing on vitamin D can only happen through man-made supplements. Just another reason to stick with the superior options Mother Nature has already provided.

Back to Nature

So take that brief midday walk in the sun. Interact with nature. It's a nice break in the day anyway, helping you manage your stress levels. And that's a good thing where vitamin D is concerned because cortisol, the "stress hormone," actually blocks the absorption of vitamin D. A nice little nature walk has multiple benefits. It reduces your stress *and* it allows the intake of a very valuable vitamin.

If you're vitamin D deficient, then why not take it seriously by dedicating some time in your day for sunshine? Make it a solid and defined part of your lifestyle. Vitamin D levels can be determined with a blood test. These levels can change dramatically over the course of just one to two months. Why not get tested before and after and see if you don't get some definitive results showing the benefits of sunshine?

Of course you don't want to get sunburned, but remember this: when you consider the way we're blocking the health forming powers of vitamin D with the toxic chemicals of sunscreen, together with the way we're compensating for our vitamin D deficiencies with man-made potentially toxic supplements, it's a safe bet that life force and longevity are compromised more by lack of sunlight than by too much. The key to getting it right is understanding how it works and striking a balance.

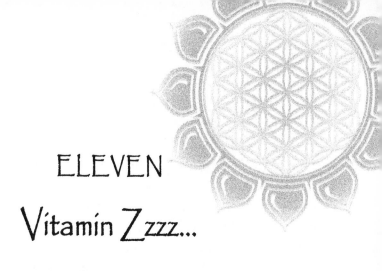

ELEVEN

Vitamin Zzzz...

We've identified how the essentials of diet, hydration and sunshine are intricately linked together. Well, here's another one: sleep! Naturally sleep has a direct impact on the performance of every function of the body, to be reflected by your energy, immune system, happiness, love-life, ability to manage stress, mental acuity, and many other things. And yet studies show that insomnia is a problem for nearly half of our population. Collectively, we're a sleep-deprived people.

So, let's figure this one out. Below are my best tips for a good night's rest:

Sleeping Environment

Consideration should be given to the bed you're sleeping on and maintaining a good bedroom environment. After all, consider we spend a significant part of our lives in bed! So what you sleep on is important. Spring beds are the most common, but they're not always without their flaws, one of them being the flame-retardant materials that they're made out of which produces toxic off-gassing. And most mattress pads are also made from petroleum products that produce similar off-gas. This wouldn't be a major concern with infrequent exposure, but, again, we're talking a substantial portion of our time spent with these pollutants.

There are beds made from natural materials, making them healthier. Beds made of natural latex are becoming much more common. That's my preference. Another option are futons consisting of purely cotton. Also sheets should be pure cotton or other natural materials, not petroleum-based polyester. And avoid blankets that are insulated with polyester too. Wash your sheets using only natural detergents. Stay away from the fragrant stuff. Again, the idea is to create a pure sleeping environment.

Cool temperatures seem to be more conducive to sleep for most people, but go with whatever makes you comfortable. I suggest cracking a window (assuming you're not living next to the interstate). After all, oxygen is the most restorative thing we put into our body. Keep things quiet. The white noise from a fan turned on low can be very effective at counteracting background noise. There are "noise machines" made specifically for the purpose of sleep. And earplugs can be an outstanding tool to thwart the common late night distractions like the neighbor's barking dog and bed mate's snoring—especially when coupled with white noise.

The darker your bedroom the better. The brain produces melatonin in dark environments, so naturally this means turn off anything that emits any light. If you have an alarm clock, make sure the display is exclusively red light. Red light is the only light that doesn't interfere with the brain's production of melatonin. Still, even if your alarm clock is red light, I suggest blocking it from your view while you're in bed. If you can see your alarm clock, you may find that you have a tendency to wake up at the same time every night. It un-instinctively trains the brain in a way most of us would not prefer. And personally when I wake up in the middle of the night, I fall back asleep much easier when I don't know what time it is. An eye mask can also be a brilliant tool if making your room very dark is not possible.

On the odd nights where you find yourself tossing and turning, it can be helpful to get up and go into another room for five minutes. It may take a moderate amount of willpower. Go pet the dog. Or throw a jacket on and go outside on your patio to get some air and take a look at the stars. Then back under the covers.

Side note: it's generally more restorative to sleep on your back and sides, rather than your stomach, at least for the majority of the night. Sleeping on your back and sides allows for deeper breathing versus sleeping on your stomach.

Sleep Supplements

What about sleep supplements? Remember that my philosophy with supplements is to use those that are exclusively from plants. Personally I've experienced little benefit with sleep supplements myself, but for some they have proven to be valuable. Sedative herbs like valerian root and kava-kava can potentially be effective sleep aides. But they *are* slightly toxic for the liver and the body's tolerance generally goes up with these herbs in just a few days. I view them as something to be used for the short term only when you really need them. Adaptogen herbs, on the other hand, simply have a calming effect on the body's nervous system. Good examples are lavender, tulsi, passionflower, and skullcap. CBD oil extracted from hemp may also be an effective option. These herbs can be taken individually or in combinations, and you'll see that many natural sleep supplements on the market are blends of several of these. These natural herbs have been utilized for thousands of years, and they can work for many people. They can be used daily, but like sedative herbs, their effectiveness tends to be reduced as tolerance goes up after a few days.

Simple chamomile tea can be another good one. Try it with a teaspoon of honey. In fact, honey alone is effective for promoting sleep. If you're making tea, try using only a little water making it concentrated to avoid the extra liquid intake for the reasons we discussed above.

The commonly known sleep supplement melatonin may be helpful in the short term, but one thing about melatonin in supplements that people don't know is that it's extracted from cow pineal glands. Yup. That's a little weird in my opinion. These are the melatonin products labeled as "natural." There are also melatonin supplements labeled as "vegan," the downside being that they're artificially lab-formulated.

Diet

Fortunately there are foods that enhance natural melatonin production in the brain. Few people know this! Bananas, pineapple, kiwi, cherries (especially tart), oats, tomatoes, rice, almonds, and goji berries. These all greatly enhance the melatonin production in the brain. On the flip side of your diet, the idea is to avoid melatonin-depleting foods. Yup, you guessed it—alcohol and sugar.

Another reason alcohol and sugar can interfere with sleep is because of the weakening effect they can have on the liver. Did you know the health of your liver can affect your sleep? This is well known in Chinese medicine and Ayurveda. Try drinking milk thistle and dandelion tea, both known to be strengthening for the liver.

Lastly, have dinner at least a few hours before going to bed. Your end of the day meal should be about getting the restorative foods: more protein, less fuel from fats and carbs. And go for easier-to-digest foods. For the late-night snack, when you need it, go for honey with a little yogurt or almond butter.

Hydration

The idea is to hydrate more during the day and less at night to keep yourself from waking up to make multiple trips to the bathroom. I generally curb my hydration after 6:00 p.m. (of course there are variable factors, like if you're out dancing late, for instance; then of course you should drink more water). Having to get up once a night is pretty common, but twice a night or more, and you may not be getting an ideal amount of uninterrupted REM (rapid eye movement) sleep. It's approximately four hours of uninterrupted REM that serves as a bit of a "reset" for the nervous system. So avoid drinking lots of fluids in the evening unless necessary and, as you'll recall from our chapter on water, this shouldn't be a problem if you're hydrating properly all day. As for caffeine, it can potentially affect the ability to sleep for up to eight hours. Plan your tea-time accordingly.

Trips to the bathroom, by the way, become a bigger problem for men than women as we get older. An enlarged prostate can lead to urinary frequency. Natural herbal supplements like saw palmetto and pumpkin seed extract (or even the whole pumpkin seeds) can be great support. Another common reason for both men and women having to make the late night trips is from blood pooling in the legs from longs days of sitting at the office. At the end of the day when the body lays flat, these stagnant fluids move around, naturally some of which is to be excreted. Try this: after work, lay flat on your back with your legs elevated for five minutes. If you're still having to make frequent trips to the bathroom, it's worth getting checked out by your doctor.

Lifestyle

Exercise! This is an important factor when it comes to getting a good night's sleep. Fatiguing your body with regular exercise will no question help you sleep better.

Naps. Cut back on long naps. Instead, try this revitalizing technique mid-day when you need it: rest ten minutes lying flat on your back. Lying flat decompresses the joints and muscles. And best of all, it puts the heart on the same level as the rest of the body, helping to re-circulate oxygen-rich blood head to toe. It will also help remedy the challenge I just mentioned above. A short rest on your back can be an outstanding pick me up and it doesn't interfere with sleep later even if you snooze a bit.

Another lifestyle factor: What are you doing in the evening? When it comes to work-related activity, try to throw in the towel at least a few hours before going to bed, giving yourself time to unwind. Keep your activity before bedtime relaxing. Take a shower, sit outside gazing at the stars, listen to your favorite (relaxing) music, talk to a friend about something that makes you happy, watch a funny movie (no drama), or read something boring (obviously that wouldn't include this exciting book!).

Keep light low in the evenings, preferably exposing yourself only to incandescent bulbs, not fluorescent. As we discussed, the brain produces more melatonin when there is less light, naturally making you better able to sleep after the sun goes down. During the evening hours reduce your time looking at back-lit screens. That means getting away from your computer—and even more importantly your smartphone since it's generally held closer to your face. Blue light emitted from screens like these reduces the production of melatonin in the brain. There are glasses made specially for filtering blue light. They may be a worthy consideration, especially if you work late at night.

Synchronize a little more with the sun if you can. Staying up late can definitely interfere with the body's natural cycles. Going to bed early and getting up early, if possible, is generally best. If waking up and not being able to fall back to sleep is typical for you, utilize a little discipline to get up earlier, spending a little less time in bed. And keep a regular sleep schedule.

Remember that, to a large degree, sleep is a function of lifestyle. All of these factors combine to affect the quality of your sleep. Take an inventory of what, in your lifestyle, is affecting your time under the covers. Examine your sleep environment. Use supplements if you have a need for them, but keep 'em natural. Natural sleep supplements are perfectly fine to use, but if you find yourself needing something more—like a valium (as any pharmaceutical, this one can potentially cause more harm than benefit)—then there's something else going on that needs to be addressed. Give it some time to get your sleep rhythms back on track. It may take a week or two, but stick with these protocols and they'll pay off. Sleep is no minor thing. Remember that it represents about a third of your life. So do it right to give your body the vitamin Z that it needs!

TWELVE

The Fundamentals of a Strong Body

We Nomads

Humans have been around for a long time but it's only been relatively recently in our history, with the development of agriculture, that we've settled ourselves into villages and, ultimately, cities. Before that, we were nomads, traveling by foot around the countryside in search of food and moving with the seasons. As a result, our bodies adapted to this kind of physical activity. Today, with our modern lifestyles, we're much less active than we previously were. We do a lot of sitting, at work, and at home. In other words, the modern way of life is not what our bodies were adapted for. This relative decline in activity can, generally speaking, result in our bodies becoming physically weaker than they really should be. And today we see the effects: a commonality of obesity and a host of other issues like heart disease.

Of course our diets are important for keeping our bodies strong. Eating healthy is a vital start. But putting fuel in is only half of it. You need to pump the handle! Human biology requires that to stay fit, we need to, at least in some way, replicate the active lifestyles of our ancestors. And that, of course, means exercise.

Extraordinary Things

Building a fit body through exercise does extraordinary things for many aspects of our overall health. Improved strength supports joints and bones and, especially, the spine. The spine, after all, is a pillar of the neurological "superhighway" through which the brain exchanges vital information with the rest of the body, and, in turn, through which the body takes care of the brain. Strong body and posture keep that superhighway healthy.

Other benefits? The obvious one is that exercise boosts our metabolism, thus reducing the amount of fat stored in the body. Leanness alone is worth the moderate effort it takes. Exercise also circulates nutrients and oxygen-rich blood to organs and every part of the body, essentially making everything stronger *and* more resistant to injury.

Furthermore, strengthening your body helps to eliminate everyday aches and pains. Your body heals faster. It's ironic, isn't it? Many people shy away from exercise *because* of aches and pains, and yet there's no better way to avoid physical discomfort in the long-term than by strengthening the body! Exercise fortifies the parts of the body around those everyday aches and pains, creating an incubating environment for the healing of the weak areas. Exercising the core can lessen back pain, for instance. The increased oxygen rich blood flow reduces inflammation so the body's restorative healing life-force can get in there to work its magic. Done properly (as we'll discuss), exercise essentially becomes physical therapy. I never stopped being amazed when I would witness this at the Ashram Health Retreat. People would experience six days of intensive exercise and leave with their everyday aches and pains gone, or at least substantially reduced.

I've experienced it firsthand myself. Years ago, I suffered from a variety of aches. Due to inflammation, I had plantar fasciitis in the arches of my feet, carpal tunnel in my wrists, and pain in my shoulders (thoracic outlet syndrome). I went to a series of specialists, some of whom recommended various surgeries. At the time I was wearing braces on my wrists and doing virtually no exercise other than limping around my living room. Finally, a doctor said something startling. "You need to take those stupid things off your wrists and get to the gym!" I took his simple advice and worked with a professional trainer and my aches and pains all went away within a few months. I didn't need surgery; I just needed to make my body stronger. The impact blew my mind. What a lesson!

Need more reasons to exercise? The data are overwhelming that exercise is a great stress-reducer—quite unlike anything else. Plus, it gives you a sense of achievement, helping to build your self-esteem. As mentioned in Chapter 10, if you exercise outside, you might even pick up some vitamin D from the sun. Not to mention that you'll pick up some peace of mind just by getting outdoors, something tried and tested for millennia.

Most people who decide they're not going to take the time to stay physically active through some kind of consistent exercise have no idea how powerful it can be and what they are missing out on. They lack the comparative experience. But for those who engage in it, they know the benefits can be enormous. Bottom line? The value of exercise is in its ability to significantly enhance life-force, longevity, and happiness. Priceless, wouldn't you say?

Aerobic and Anaerobic

As many of us know, there are two general categories of exercise: aerobic, also known as "cardio," and anaerobic which is generally load-bearing or the expenditure of energy in bursts, like sprints. You need to get the heart rate up with sustained aerobic activity, but you need to build muscle via anaerobic activity, too. By building muscle with load-bearing exercise, your body naturally burns more calories on a consistent basis. You're building a bigger engine which requires more fuel! So the priority isn't necessarily losing weight, it's building strength which produces a leaner body.

There's one particular exercise that, for the money, is the most efficient in combining both cardio and load-bearing activity: hiking. After all, trekking up and down hills is just what our ancestors did. The distances we are capable of hiking are commonly underestimated. During the one-week program at the Ashram, we'd hike with the guests ten to fifteen miles a day for seven days straight! And not everyone was always the most fit. But again, hiking this kind of mileage is what we are adapted to do.

Of course, generally speaking, we don't have the time to hike for hours every day. But even going a few miles at a sturdy pace two or three days per week can have a tremendous impact. You're getting your heart rate up *and* lifting your body weight as you trek up and down hills, making hiking the perfect cardio and load-bearing activity, all in one. Plus, you're exercising the largest muscles in your body— namely your gluteus muscles and quads in your legs—which therefore has the most effect on your metabolism. And you're strengthening your core, too. When you're hiking over uneven terrain, you're also exercising your smaller, stabilizer muscles—lots of little muscles that all add up. There's a *lot* you can cover by just walking up and down hills.

Popular ways that people try to replicate this kind of physical activity are in the gym via stationary bikes or treadmills. These are obviously much better alternatives than not exercising at all. But when doing only the same repetitive motion that's offered by stationary bikes or treadmills, you can't really get the same kind of workout provided by hiking and navigating hills. Essentially, all of those stabilizer muscles aren't really working. And, you're not getting outside which is always the place I prefer to do at least a portion of my exercise. Do you live somewhere flat? No worries. A brisk walk, followed by doing a few sets of squats while holding a dumbbell to your chest, qualifies as an awesome workout.

As for load-bearing exercise, remember that the gluteus muscles and quads should be your highest priority for enhancing your metabolism and building your overall strength. The seldom-done squats and deadlifts are hands down the best gym exercises you can do because of the emphasis on these bigger muscles as well as your core strength. Deadlifts have an undeserved negative reputation (the name doesn't help—better would be "life-lifts" or "anti-death lifts"!) that comes from too many people doing them inappropriately, with too much weight and with the wrong form. Just like hiking, bending over or squatting to pick up heavy objects is something humans have been doing for quite some time; thus our bodies are well adapted to do these exercises. But don't risk an injury. Do them right. Your best bet? Work with the theme "less weight, more reps." Also these lifting exercises don't necessarily need to be committed to with a bar. Using dumbbells or kettle-bells is a great, low-risk way to get started. Rubber exercise bands can be excellent tools as well. And why not work with a trainer? I do, and I can't recommend it highly enough!

Remember to maintain stretching as a part of your physical activity. Maintaining elasticity of muscles is vital for a whole host of reasons, the most important of which is prevention of injury, inflammation, and those everyday aches and pains. It's important for maintaining good posture, too. A full body stretch doesn't need to take more than a few minutes. Actually, a common mistake can be *over*-stretching, which can make muscles weaker. Of course muscles can be re-strengthened, but why put your body through unnecessary stress? If you choose a yoga practice, the idea is to hold the stretching poses for only seconds. It's the *strengthening* poses that can be held for longer. There is some reasoning however for holding the stretching poses longer, and it's for the releasing of deeper tension. So in a sense there can be a benefit to this. My suggestion if you do the longer stretching poses is to do them only on an occasional basis, especially if building strength is what you're going for.

While we're on the subject of stretching, here's an oft-over-looked part of the body you should definitely make it a point to stretch: your arches! In a way, our feet are a foundational element. Taking care of them is reflected throughout the body. The key is to spend at least *some* time on your bare feet. Around the house, for instance. Arches are your body's natural suspension, vastly better than the foam cushioning you find in shoes with arch support (the role these shoes can fulfill is running on pavement, but are needed for little else). Going barefoot stretches out the arches and stretching anything means getting oxygen-rich blood to the areas that need it.

I learned this the hard way from my experience with plantar fasciitis. I was told I needed arch support and so I bought expensive ones, wanting to make sure I had the best available. By then, the pain was so bad that it hurt to walk anywhere and, consequently, I did very little of it. Thinking I was better supporting my arches, I wore shoes all the time, right up to the moment I got into bed each night. Turns out, just like with the wrist braces, I was doing the exact opposite of what I should have been doing. On a camping trip, my shoes got so muddy one day that I had no choice but to take them off and walk around barefoot. And a funny thing happened. My pain went away almost immediately. Why? Because I was stretching my arches out. Just another example of how the body can heal naturally if we just let it.

Speaking of going barefoot in the great outdoors, did you know that there is an electrical current in the ground? Now consider the fact that, to a very real extent, our bodies are finely-tuned electrical organisms—the brain, heart, and nerves being prime examples. Internally, there are conductive systems that deliver necessary electrons throughout all parts of the body for the purpose of neutralizing otherwise harmful free radicals. These important electrons are the very same electrons that we have the potential to absorb from the bare ground into our feet. This is perhaps one of the reasons walking barefoot at the beach is a common favorite. Conduction of these electrons into our feet is effective only on bare ground. Concrete (not asphalt) and brick are the exceptions. Today, because we are generally wearing rubber-soled shoes, we are missing out on this natural grounding effect. There's plenty of data to support this, so do yourself a favor and spend a little time outside on your bare feet.

Hire a Pro

As mentioned, I highly recommend working with a fitness trainer. What you learned in PE class in high school about exercise just isn't going to cut it. And going to the gym on your own and doing the same routine day in and day out only does so much. It's much more effective and time better spent to shake things up. The variety of fitness activities is endless, and changing up the exercises you're doing on a regular basis will make you stronger faster. A trainer knows best how to do this.

Find a trainer who believes in sticking with the free weights. Free weights have exponentially more impact than machines. Remember that core and lower-body exercises are the most important since, as we discussed above, they're the biggest muscles. Men especially tend to get preoccupied with upper body workouts, partly because they're easier overall since the upper body muscles are smaller relative to the muscles in the legs. It's a matter of balance between lower and upper-body exercises, but placing more of an emphasis on lower-body is the way to go. And of course we're not talking body-building here. We're talking about strength and life-force building.

In my mind, working with a professional trainer is one of the very best ways you can spend your money, right up there with diet. When you think about how much we spend on educating our minds in school, working with a trainer is a small price to pay for improving the body (which improves the mind, too!) In the end, it's an extremely cost-effective way to build and enhance your health. And it needn't be time-consuming. With the right kind of intensive exercise, you can get a lot out of a single hour, or even less. Believe me, I've seen the results firsthand through trainers I have worked with, and by my own experience as a trainer at the Ashram. I've witnessed incredible transformations in people of all body types and starting out at all different levels of fitness.

Keep in mind you don't have to work with a trainer every day. Why not start with just two days a week? Of course a good trainer will teach you how to work out on your own, too. I'm confident you'll be very impressed with what you get out of it.

The other days of the week? Hike or go for power walks! I am very much a believer in fast-paced walking. Too easy for you? Try carrying five or ten pound dumbbells (or water bottles) and pump your arms like you mean it. Now we're talking. Or maybe you've got other athletic pursuits—sports that you like to play. Being physically active should be enjoyable, something you look forward to. Yoga, soccer, pottery (well maybe something a little more strenuous), swimming, and biking—they're all good. Need I share my opinion of the contact sports like football that invite injury and wear and tear on the body? Get creative. Join a softball team. Take up tennis. Play ultimate Frisbee. Dance! (This one is among my favorites, on which I'll elaborate in Chapter 14.) Hey, want a good workout? Ratchet up the times you're intimate with your partner. Seriously! You'll notice an increase in stamina there, as well. Do it for health. And for love of course.

Exercise is certainly neck and neck with diet, in terms of importance for overall health. They're both critical links in the chain of well-being. Remember that when we neglect our diets, we lose the energy and enthusiasm we need to be physically active. It becomes hard to exercise even if we want to. So create the right chemistry with your diet and then pump the handle with exercise. And don't forget that your mental well-being is connected directly to your physiological health. No question a strong body is one of the foundational elements for a strong mind, only to make us more fit to better navigate through the world of modern stressors. Even giving yourself just a few hours a week will have tremendous payoff.

THIRTEEN

Disease Prevention and Healing

Everything we've discussed so far relates to nothing less than building life-force. Diet, exercise, hydration, even sunshine and sleep—it's all connected. And one of the great results of living a healthy way of life? Taken care of properly, your body is less likely to experience illness and physical distress. By maximizing those things that strengthen the body and minimizing the things that weaken the body, naturally you'll be able to enjoy life at your greatest potential. And vulnerability to ailments of any sort will be substantially reduced.

I'm not claiming that you'll never fall ill or be victim to disease. But I can state with confidence that your odds will be lower as your body's healing powers become greater. The body is commonly underestimated when it comes to both prevention and healing. We live in a society where often the first recourse is to turn to modern science, to depend on pharmaceuticals or surgeries to fix what's ailing us. But a body well taken care of has an extraordinary ability to take care of itself, and even heal itself. Life-force created via lifestyle heals and is the body's preferred remedy.

The lifestyle I advocate in this book can be thought of as a "medicinal" lifestyle. When we take care of the body, we help prevent disease. And if and when we get sick, symptoms can be minimized and recovery can be faster. I know from my own experience. My brain condition which I spoke of in the Introduction is partly genetic. It's been a terrible privilege. It has forced me into a much more serious look at my lifestyle, and, in fact, a more serious look at the Western lifestyle in general. And the adjustments I've made in my life have all had a payoff greater than I would have ever expected. The potential for miraculous healing is built inside us. Eliminating the common stressors from our diet and lifestyle makes way for this reality to show itself.

There are, of course, thousands of diseases and I can't elaborate on specific curatives. There are volumes upon volumes of information out there about the many maladies that exist and the potential natural treatments. But in looking at the big picture, we can accurately say this about disease prevention and healing: it boils down to maintaining a strong heart, strong digestive and immune systems, and a healthy brain. And naturally these are interconnected, along with everything else in the body. Everything we do either makes these pillars weaker or stronger.

Let's also look as this on the cellular level since cells are what everything in our bodies is made of. Cells operate under a simple process of uptaking oxygen, glucose, and water and then eliminating waste. The idea is to give them healthy fuel, hydration, and an environment free of stagnant adrenaline from stress and of course free of toxins from a polluted diet and lifestyle. Essentially, any one of these unhealthy stressors interferes with a cell's function. First thing compromised is waste elimination which reduces its uptake of adequate oxygen and glucose. This makes the cell weaker which then compromises the strength of every organ and function in the body.

This is why maintaining the perspective of replacing the elements in our day to day lives that incur wear and tear with those that are restorative is so valuable. The body's primary healing agent is oxygen and nutrient-rich blood that we create with our diet and lifestyle which we have defined throughout this book. There are a few essentials for enabling your heart to pump that healing agent throughout the body in order to get to each and every cell. Here is where it's vitally important to understand that it's free radicals that cause the most interference with this process. Free radicals are molecules that are unstable due to missing electrons. These unstable molecules travel through the body creating wear and tear and, in particular, inflammation, thus inhibiting the free flow of nutrient-rich blood. Now remember in the exercise chapter I talked about how free electrons from the bare ground have the potential to play a big role here. Free electrons link with free radicals making them stable again, to then become a properly functioning molecule. And here is exactly where antioxidants meet this vital need, too. Antioxidants lend these very same free electrons. And what's the primary source? Raw fruits and vegetables! The first thing is getting the free radical-causing toxins out of the way with a cleaner diet and lifestyle. Moderate amounts of free radicals are actually part of just simple day to day living. Counteracting this normal amount is no problem for the body when living a healthy lifestyle. But toxins such as sugar and cooked unsaturated fats (especially fried food) in our diet, stress, and over-exposure to the sun are a few examples of what can significantly expedite the production of these damaging free radicals. So, plain and simple, the main idea is to replace the destructive elements with the restorative. And then pump that handle with exercise to get the antioxidants circulated throughout the body in order to stabilize molecules and reduce inflammation so nutrient rich blood can get to each and every cell to work its restorative magic. Make sense?

Keeping this simple concept in mind helps put things in perspective, hopefully to influence better decision making with diet and lifestyle. After all, knowing *why* you're doing the healthy things you're doing is a much more effective way for helping stay on track than doing things strictly out of discipline. It's another case of discipline shifting to desire. And that's what paves the way for a lifestyle that lasts a lifetime.

Cancer and Heart Disease

Of all the diseases, cancer and heart disease are statistically the most fatal in the Western world. As for cancer, we're in a much better position today than yesterday, at least from an informational standpoint. We've identified many of the causes, like smoking and toxic chemicals and processed sugar. The key, therefore, is knowledge. We've learned it's often about going after the cause rather than the symptom.

Naturally there are no sure-things, but being informed and living a healthier lifestyle can certainly increase our chances of cancer prevention. And recovery, if need be. Whether it's prevention or healing, it's really all about strengthening the immune system. We've talked at length about detoxifying your diet and living environment, removing the causatives of mis-programmed cells in your body. There are a few key additions that should be more commonly known like adding more foods high in vitamin C. Vitamin C (one of those essential antioxidants) is an amazing immune-system booster, reputed to be the most effective anti-cancer agent there is. Don't forget, also, that vitamin D is a huge part of your immune system. It's quite an irony that the correct amount of sunshine for vitamin D has proven to help with cancer recovery. (Remember, of course, that too much sun can have the opposite effect.) And besides getting sunshine, spending time outside in the wonders of nature has a brilliant effect on the mind which plays a definite role in prevention of ailments such as cancer. (Stay tuned, we'll talk more about the role of the mind in healing and some notes on how to strengthen it in the next chapter.)

As for heart disease, the prevalence is on the rise. Here again, we know the answers. Reduce saturated fat—most importantly, low-quality animal protein and hydrogenated vegetable oils. Decrease your stress levels. Exercise more often to strengthen your heart.

Even still, life comes with no guarantees. If you're fighting cancer or heart disease, you might consider going full-court press, taking advantage of what modern medicine can do for you, but no doubt whilst living a healing lifestyle. It's a two-pronged attack. My feelings about Western medicine are admittedly mixed. I'm often amazed by what science has discovered yet I find myself disturbed by the pervasiveness of pharmaceuticals that are prescribed for even just minor infections. And we all know that, due to common side effects, they can sometimes cause more harm than benefit.

I humbly admit that seizure medicine has played a very important role in my life. I learned the hard way that stubbornly going medication-free wasn't worth the grand-mal seizures that would involve being unconscious and biting the heck out of my tongue. Unfortunately the common seizure meds are known to have some of the worst of side effects. Now of course this was *not* reason to throw in the towel on living the medicinal lifestyle! Quite the contrary. Rather it's *more* of a reason to live a healthy life to reduce a medication's side effects by supporting the liver, kidneys, digestion, and the other detoxifying elements in the body. Also I did the extensive research to find the medication that had the *least* side effects of the many options. The one I chose actually doesn't stop the seizure from happening. Rather it keeps it from becoming severe. The upside of this was that I have been able to gauge what it was in my lifestyle that would help prevent the seizure from happening in the first place. What a valuable opportunity.

It is worth noting the natural supplements—medicinal herbs—can provide at least some degree of support for virtually any malady. They have for me. There are literally thousands of medicinal herbs that have tons of data supporting their effectiveness but are lesser known by modern doctors. Between Western Herbology, Naturopathy, Chinese medicine, and Ayurvedic medicine, there are excellent and even potentially superior alternatives to Western medicine. I view the mastery of medical doctors to be the diagnosing and the mastery of naturopaths (and similar) to be the healing. I'm very much a believer in the variety of other healing modalities including acupuncture, massage, aromatherapy, reiki, reflexology, and more. I believe in prayer too, which we'll talk about in the next chapter.

THE INFINITY HEALTH MANUAL

Of course each person will have to decide the best way to treat their own ailments. But the means of disease prevention and healing provided by natural alternatives are on the rise and can all play a big role with the treatment of any and every ailment. Meet with a naturopath and other healers to take advantage of what's out there and discover the potential curatives that would be the most fitting for you, if and when you need them. But don't forget that no matter what route you take, a healthy lifestyle remains your best bet.

Autoimmune Disease

The most common disease of our modern world, yet ironically the least-understood, is autoimmune disease. Autoimmune disease affects at least *twenty-five million* people in the United States. That's eight percent of our population. And it's rapidly increasing. In comparison, cancer affects nine million and heart disease affects twenty-two million. And yet, autoimmune disease is the disease most Americans seem to be least aware of. So what the heck is it?

First, although it's often confused with AIDS, the two are completely different. AIDS, of course, is a transmitted virus that attacks the immune system. Autoimmune disease is when the immune system turns on and attacks the body itself. Essentially, the immune system gets a mind of its own and goes after its own organs. This is something that is often brought on by an unhealthy lifestyle and is *not* transmittable between individuals.

Just forty years ago, autoimmune disease was virtually non-existent. Interestingly, in third-world countries, it's still virtually non-existent. It exists almost exclusively in developed countries. So what's going on? While we don't need to fear autoimmune disease, we do need to educate ourselves about it. Essentially, we need to pay attention to the basic facts and adjust our lifestyles accordingly.

There are around a hundred known strains of autoimmune disease and more are coming out all the time. Besides allergies (the most common affliction of autoimmune disease), some of the more well-known strains include type-1 diabetes, rheumatoid arthritis, lupus, multiple sclerosis, thyroid disease, asthma, eczema, inflammatory bowel disease, psoriasis, and celiac disease. The common denominator is the attack of the body by the immune system. Psoriasis, for example, is the immune system attacking the skin. Rheumatoid arthritis is the immune system attacking the joints. Multiple sclerosis is the immune system attacking the brain. The most common effect on the attacked area of the body is inflammation, the swelling of tissues, making it unreachable for nutrient rich blood that is trying to come to the rescue.

Is There a Solution for Autoimmune Disease?

The most commonly used medical "solution" for autoimmune disease is, not surprisingly, Western medication. As I explained, medication may not always be all bad, and, more often than not, autoimmune disease medications can relieve the symptoms. Unfortunately, these medications are among the most severe in terms of their side effects. Their intent is to suppress the immune system and weaken its attack on the body. It's a bit like trying to clear the smoke out of your house rather than putting out the fire, a temporary solution that allows you to catch your breath at best. In the world of autoimmune disease, medication should ideally be considered a short-term solution, or at least only part of it.

Autoimmune disease is greatly correlated with diet and lifestyle—often more so than most other diseases. The aim is to cool the inflammation, which boils down to finding the source. Here is where we need to address the cause more than the symptom. Some autoimmune diseases are genetic but they can still be exacerbated by one's lifestyle. What is it in the diet or lifestyle of the person living with an autoimmune disorder that is wreaking the havoc? Although that can be difficult to identify, the good news is that that is actually one of the specialties of natural medicine. There are numerous cases of autoimmune disease being healed in the realm of functional, holistic, and alternative medicine. This is where medicinal herbs can play a tremendous role, and I would encourage you to find yourself a trained, certified herbalist to walk you through the many available options.

With autoimmune disease, the overall key is take hold of the reins of the out-of-control immune system. Essentially, it's like an untrained mustang bucking and kicking. We don't want to abandon the horse altogether; we just want to tame it. The immune system works hand in hand with the neurological system that extends throughout the body. Mostly it's about adding vital nutrients that recover the intelligence of the immune system while cutting the toxic junk out. Believe it or not, adding a few things to your diet and removing a few others is what most often saves the day. This is where a food allergy test could be invaluable. And remember there are two nutrients that are the most important: vitamin C and vitamin D (a common theme, right?).

Some might think boosting the immune system (which these vitamins are known for) would be the exact wrong thing to do, given the fact that the immune system is already attacking itself. But what you're really doing is restoring your body's instinctive healing wisdom. The intelligence of the immune system is awesome, and it does a lot more than just fighting colds.

Again, for the sake of your body's healing powers it's vital to cut out the junk. By now, you can guess what the food culprits are: processed sugar, low-grade animal protein, cheap oils, flour, and similar heavily processed food. Another huge "junk" factor is toxic chemicals. We talked about these earlier. Toxic household items like cleaners and air-fresheners are proven to exacerbate autoimmune disease. Unquestionably, these can be original causatives, at least to some degree, and over time the wear and tear of these pollutants weakens the immune system.

Another culprit: antibacterial soap and hand sanitizers are taking on the role of your immune system and doing a much worse job. In December of 2013, the FDA proposed questioning soap companies to address the potential risks of using such products daily. The active antibacterial ingredient has been proven to be toxic, and on top of this, there's no evidence that antibacterial soap products are any more effective at preventing illness than washing with plain soap and water. Finally, as of this writing, it looks as though the FDA is going to ban these terrible soaps. Let the immune system do its job!

Something else: antibiotics and some vaccines are now linked to autoimmune disease. The data are real. These culprits kill the bad bacteria while also killing the good bacteria we need in order to maintain a healthy immune system. Antibiotics may be used when the situation is desperate and life threatening. Even still, once utilized, there needs to be some follow-up damage control with a healing diet and lifestyle. Most important is replacing the intestinal flora that gets killed with the use of antibiotics. This is the role of a probiotic supplement.

It should be noted here that for some people living with an autoimmune disease, one-hundred percent healing may not always happen. But at the very least, the symptoms can be reduced and may eventually go away entirely. There have been many cases where toxic foods were identified and removed, ultimately letting the body heal itself. These stories point us in a very clear direction.

With regard to any malady, a medicinal lifestyle cannot be emphasized enough. The potential healing powers of the body are awesome. All we need to do is nurture it with diet, exercise, pure water, fresh air, and sunshine. And positive thinking, too! Maintain a strong heart, strong digestive and immune systems, and a healthy brain. The magnificent life-force this can yield is the body's preferred remedy.

FOURTEEN

The Power of the Mind

The Mind-Body Connection

It's interesting to contemplate that a significant purpose of keeping your body healthy is to best take care of your brain. In turn, your brain reciprocates by taking better care of your body. It's the brain that tells the body how to function and tells the organs what to do. The neurological system truly is the core of our health. All that we've talked about in this book is correlated with the idea that *everything* works better with a healthy neurological system.

Let's also consider that a healthy neurological system supports and enhances our sense of peace and happiness, as well as our memory and awareness. It makes us nicer, too! Less irritable and grouchy for sure. And much better able to cope with the stresses of everyday life. Essentially, the brain is the seat of the mind—your very self. Let a strong, healthy mind be a motivating factor behind keeping a healthy body. Sturdy connection between your internal facets is an invaluable theme to bear in mind.

As for what defines a healthy mind, let me say that I'm presenting my thoughts here with a lot of humility. I don't pretend to have all of life's answers. I see my perspective on life and the universe as just a tiny drop of water in an endless ocean of knowledge. There are many brilliant philosophical minds that have pondered the mysteries of life going back thousands of years. Yours included! No question you have a unique message about reality, making you an irreplaceable wealth of knowledge.

For me, it was when I was in the midst of the brain condition which I described in the Introduction that I found myself contemplating life, and what's behind it, as never before. Nothing focuses the mind quite like the sudden realization of life's brevity. There was one specific year within my healing journey in which I struggled especially hard with my condition. Significant bleeding in my brain caused even more seizures. Sometimes even the entire left side of my body would go numb. The whole experience dramatically shifted my attention. Mostly, it shifted my attention away from all the smaller day-to-day worries like work, money, running errands, where I needed to be, etc. In a sense, my condition was, ironically, stress-reducing!

Breathing & Meditation

During this period, I spent much more of my time outdoors in stillness and quiet. One thing that played an especially large role for me with gaining a deeper peace of mind was the practice of improving my breathing. The extraordinary healing and restorative powers of oxygen can be easy to forget. If it sounds simple, that's because it is. It's something we all instinctively know, yet underestimate. I highly recommend taking some time each day, preferably early, to sit quietly and practice your breathing. Make it a part of your daily lifestyle.

Purposeful breathing has the effect of training your body to breathe correctly, even in times of stress. Under stress, breathing becomes relatively shallow. Nevertheless, your brain is like a muscle, with muscle memory. Practice on a daily basis and your brain will respond. You'll breathe better all day long, helping you maintain a more peaceful, less-stressful frame of mind—and stronger body, too. And let's look at it from a purely physiological standpoint. Oxygen is the most essential life-support we know. We can go for days without water. Without food, a few weeks. Without oxygen, we can only go for a minute or two. Upping our intake of this vital element has an influence on our health and life-force unlike anything else. Deep breathing has even been proven to lower blood pressure! That's a big deal and very much worth our attention. (It's interesting to ponder the idea that the subtler things in life like the air we breathe, things that can't be seen, heard, or felt, are yet among the most profound. I take this as a brilliant message from the universe.)

A tip to significantly increase effectiveness of this practice: relax your lower abdomen and gently let it expand out as you inhale—we're talking the belly rather than the chest. Then fill your chest after your belly. Think of it as filling your lungs from the bottom up. This is commonly referred to as diaphragmatic breathing. You can actually increase the volume of your lung space by fifty percent with this simple technique! And now you're using your diaphragm to breathe, like the body naturally did before the commonality of modern day stress.

During this practice breathe through your nose. This by nature is the body's preferred way to breathe. The nasal pathway filters and balances the moisture of the air, optimizing it for maximum absorption in the lungs. Note: if your nose is often blocked, then lay off wheat and dairy for a couple weeks. Try to keep your living environment as low-dust as possible. If this doesn't help then get an allergy test. And experiment with a neti-pot which has proven to be an effective remedy in Ayurvedic medicine for millennia. As for the pace of your breath, relax and let your body breathe at the rate it wishes. This is part of your body's wisdom and you can trust it. There are many breathing exercises which can offer great meditative experiences, but this is the one that really does the trick for training the body and is beneficial for anyone to practice. This is essentially going straight to the finish line and breathing exactly the way the body is meant to.

Take note of how you're breathing right now, and give this a shot for just a minute. In doing this, you'll not only be saturating your bloodstream with valuable oxygen, you'll be mobilizing stale blood from organs and expelling built-up carbon dioxide from the body. You'll also be retraining yourself in proper breathing, resynchronizing this vital process. You'll end up breathing more oxygen throughout the day, making this one of the best things you can do for yourself. And it's one that's easy to get into the habit of doing. For me, it's become a very joyous part of my day. I suggest devoting at least ten minutes daily to this practice.

The setting with this plays a significant role. Create a quiet environment free of stimulation, although some soft background music is okay. Just be sure it's uplifting. I almost always couple this practice with time outdoors, typically early in the morning. Nature is a powerful force for the mind. Sit tall and hold your spine erect. Seated in a chair is fine but on the ground is better. Sitting on a cushion so your pelvis is higher off the ground than the knees will be helpful for maintaining a good posture. If sitting this way feels uncomfortable, try it for a few days and it will quickly feel more natural. After all, this is the way we were born to sit. As for what to think about, that's up to you, but the aim is to keep it positive. Even better is to allow the mind to relax and be still. This happens naturally when focusing on abdominal breathing. Remember in the chapter about digestion I explained how the majority of the body's serotonin resides in the gut. It's the reason that the notion of "using your gut instinct" has some legitimate truth to it and is also why this practice is largely about tuning in to a different layer of our consciousness from the thinking mind. I do believe this strengthens the intuitive senses, such as when to go right and when to go left. The value of this is tremendous. (We'll delve further into this topic in my next book!)

A gentle smile throughout this practice helps enrich the mood of the experience. You may not have moments of ecstatic revelation (although you may!), but you will be training your mind and body to become better fit to receive positive inspiration throughout the day. I've taken to keeping a journal for thoughts that come to me through my quiet moments. Occasionally I read through old journals, and often I'm surprised by the valuable content I had written even years before. It seems to help make such material more familiar in my everyday thought.

During times of practiced stillness, I work to contemplate the things I'm grateful for. Gratitude is a practice of rewriting a better script in your consciousness. I liken gratitude to a breeze on a flame inside us. In my daily journal I record at least two things that I am feeling grateful for. I recommend doing this. It's a proven means of making us happier. I also see it as a way of clearing the cobwebs to connect with a more steadfast sense of appreciation that life is truly brilliant. And like everything else, a feeling of gratitude is something that can become stronger, especially when making it part of a daily practice.

There's another meditative technique of simply standing tall. All it involves is standing with your feet at shoulder width, spine erect, shoulders back, and chin up with your gaze fixed on the horizon. And, as with a sitting meditation, wear a gentle smile. Your hands can be positioned however you prefer, but I like placing my hands on my hips. It's somewhat of a "superhero" posture. Let's call it "the poise of power." If this stance doesn't match your mood then it's a good reason to do it. It's essentially taking the concept of "fake it till you make it" up a level to "practice it till you become it." Modern psychology has proven that the body performs as a compass for the mind. From a metaphysical sense, healthful postures can serve as an antenna for the mind. This is part of the philosophy behind yoga. The word yoga means "unify." Ancient yoga came from the philosophy that holding specific postures opens the way for the consciousness to connect with and receive divine energies. And such influences as lengthening of hamstrings were just side-effects, as great as they were.

As part of your meditative practice, I feel the need to emphasize once again the benefit of spending at least some of this time in beautiful places outdoors, the setting being a significant element for our state of mind. Mountains, oceans, canyons, and sunsets. They're restorative nutrition for the consciousness. They can support us in ways nothing else can. If you live in an urban environment, make time for a weekend drive out into the country to enjoy the natural elements. And visit your local park. Often! Take a blanket, your journal, and a thermos of chai, known for millennia to be an ancient elixir of the soul. And spend some time barefoot! This is all restorative for the human spirit, and is, in my opinion, among the best therapies, especially with that hot drink in hand.

Make some time in your life for the meditative moments of quiet. I'm confident you will gain something from it. Our minds weren't designed to spend their time caught up in today's busy world. In a culture of unhealthy products and entertainment, it's a challenge to not fall victim to the spells of mass-distraction that modern media can put upon us. For the sake of protecting our consciousness from weakening stimulation, let's steer clear of the propaganda that brings us down or lures us into anything unhealthy. Rather, let's dedicate some time each day to non-stimulation and self-reflection. In the stillness, there's a special magic to be found that cleanses the mind and resets our attraction toward the better things in life.

A Larger Perspective

I believe that deep in the mind we all have an intuitive knowing that there's an unwavering excellence to the universe and our place in it. We can see perfection from the micro scale of the atom, up to the grand cosmic scale of the stars and galaxies. I see us as the link where the two meet. We're a part of it. We're in this universe, and this universe is in *us*. Today, the thread of perfection inside us can often be easy to forget, making a good reason for taking the time to step back and quietly contemplate our place in the cosmos. I've found that working to maintain this perspective gives a sense of being connected with a greater source of life. Why not call it a metaphysical sense? Naturally, the question arises: could there be a consciousness behind it all? An invisible hand involved with everything that we do? A God? This is something that I approach with deep humility. In the past, my faith has wavered as my boat has been rocked over the years. It's a question that I pray about daily. My wish with all of this is very much to have a clearer sense of a Great Spirit. What a wonderful thing that we are on this path of discovery together. If you feel called, why not choose a spiritual practice—yoga, qigong, shamanism, or a religion— something that resonates with your soul. Honestly, I'm partially reluctant to suggest religion since many of them argue with each other, the irony being that they are all trying to get to the same place. But any religion that influences its people to become nicer and more understanding toward *everyone*, regardless of ethnicity or religion, has my appreciation. The main criteria to search for are finding a path that reveals to you a deeper sense of your strength and joy, and a genuine wish for the same in others.

Nevertheless, I believe that we ourselves have metaphysical powers that can override the apparent limitations of the physical world. We are so much more than seemingly limited minds and bodies. The fabric of reality has proven to be malleable depending on the activity behind the eyes of the beholder. I work to view life in the context of participation with the unlimited. The fact is, we are derivatives of an imperishable universe of infinite possibility. Faith within this frame of thought can be an antidote for developing a deeper sense of faith in ourselves. It can be a means of dissipating the veils of self-doubt and fear, making us better able to see our lives rich with capability and magic. This sense is the part of ourselves that is also able to help us during times of fear, grieving, heartbreak, illness, pain, and other trials in life. This is not to say we can bandage all of life's problems with light. Nor is it always easy to find this ability in ourselves. For me, a sense of this selfhood can become out of reach during the toughest moments. This is where the love from friends and family can demonstrate its healing powers. For the same reason, we're here for our friends and family. But also deep inside there is a place we can be held in repose that can carry us along the journey of healing and restoration. The view that I work to maintain during these periods of feeling stretched and cracked, is that ripples from the challenge travel out to then be received down the road as waves of new wisdom and power. It is then that our problems become relatively smaller as our strength becomes greater.

The Greatest Element

The programming of the heart defines the greatest treasure in life to be love. It's the iridescent diamond of the Universe—all the way from true romance to the love for family and friends. After all, it's from where we all have come. Extending love toward others (strangers included), through acts and words of kindness is what makes us happier and stronger. It makes those others happier and stronger, too. Loving affection is an unparalleled remedy for both the giver and receiver. More love in our community can begin with us. Cultivation of genuine, non-egotist love is a lifelong journey we are all on together. Have faith in yourself that you are on this path. Love's extraordinary powers make it the ultimate medicine for the human spirit of which we are all a vital part. I believe that there will be a day when the willfulness to harm will be wiped away from our planet by this very force, including every bullet to battleship, to make way for greater expression of our enlightened nature. I daresay this time is not distant. May the world come home to this place in its consciousness. Our genes are programmed to know that kindness unveils a special joy unlike anything else. Carrying forward in our day-to-day lives from the perspective of service and looking out for one another brings a sense of satisfaction unlike anything else. Also within this way of thought comes a refined sense of our unique abilities of how to make the world a better place, as well as the powers around us from which we are becoming more fit to receive. Essentially, the universe is looking to express its power and intelligence by means of you. And *you* are one of a kind that can support humanity in ways that no one else can.

While we're on this subject, think about just who it is you're spending your time with. Do they make you happy or bring you down? And are you making *them* happy? Cultivate a lifestyle that for much of the time surrounds yourself with positive people you truly enjoy. But have patience with others that you come across in life that aren't quite there. Remember that we all get stressed out from time to time and if you find yourself on the receiving end of someone's negativity, it might just be that they're having a bad hair day. Do your best to not take it personally. "Blessed are the peacemakers." Let that be *you*.

Remedy of Forgiveness

This is an act of kindness that helps *you* as much as the person you need to forgive. We've all experienced grudges to be profoundly unhealthy. Thankfully, we're built with the capacity to forgive. It's the expertise of our hearts. And hey, don't forget to forgive yourself, too. It's not healthy to go around being your own worst critic. How we think about ourselves and life on earth is equally, if not more, important than diet (the good news is the two work hand in hand).

Self Esteem

This brings up the topic of self-esteem. We all have our challenging periods of criticizing our own weaknesses. Negative thoughts about ourselves do not have to hang over our consciousness. Viewing thoughts of self-criticism and worry as passing clouds is a practice. A reality to be considered is that it's the weak places in us that are also where we have the greatest potential to grow. The big questions to ask ourselves are: "What are my strengths?" (Having trouble of thinking of any? Ask a friend.) And "How can my strengths support the weaknesses?" The answers to these questions can help clear the way for a new view of your previously underestimated positive qualities. And here is another concept to practice—choose to make happiness a cause in life rather than waiting for it as an effect. It's a natural ability of the human spirit and is something I work on in my practice every day.

I also work to remember that periods of feeling weak or down are only temporary, and the growing that takes place throughout these times has the potential to yield a tremendous esteem-building sense of achievement. It's the nature of personal growth—a course of action that never ends. Building self-esteem and casting aside shame and similar types of stagnation is a life journey we are all on together. Thankfully, for all of us, the feeble myth of an undeserved guilt is a dying paradigm. Rather we are living a way of life dedicated to clearing the path for a steadfast sense of joy to be a more permanent trait of our consciousness, rather than a temporary state of the mind—both for our own wellbeing as well as for the wellbeing of those whom we influence. By the way, this is part of why I have given up the use of mind altering substances, the aim being an achievement of *longer-lasting* "substances" such as self-esteem and happiness. Lastly, I can assure you that incorporating the healthful information we have discussed throughout this book plays a tremendous role in how we feel about ourselves, our joy, and our overall mental wellbeing. And vice-versa! A healthy mind supports living a more intelligible way of life. The wellbeing between mind and body is a brilliant synergy.

Awe

Awe is a quality of mind that I've experienced to have great value when maintained in my daily thought. Marveling at the expanse of reality, the universe, and our place in it can provide a powerful state of mind to be in, and there are ways to stir it up. One of my favorite ways is to ponder, especially outside at night while gazing at the stars, the unimaginable vastness of the universe. Consider that the nearest star, Proximus Centauri, is four light-years away. This means that it takes four years for light from this star to reach us. And light travels at 700 million miles per hour. Here's a mathematical way to put that into perspective (and to me this one never gets old): the fastest humans have ever traveled is 25,000 miles per hour in a space shuttle entering our atmosphere. That's fast! If we were to travel that fast towards Proximus Centauri, it would take 112,000 years to get there. Now think about this: the farthest stars we've identified are over *fifty million* light years away! Want more to ponder? Think of what's beyond *those* stars. Now compare such miracles to our very selves. Fundamentally we are time-traveling emanations from the beginning of the universe, alive and infused with majesty, order, and intelligence. Awe—I consider it an invaluable state of mind that we can readily stir into action. It's a capacity that arouses receptors in our consciousness for the mystical and magical, to be discovered and strengthened by *you*.

The Magic of Dance

On the quest to connect with ourselves, the universe, and the moment, there's a tried and true practice that goes back to the ancients: dance. Dance is a significant part of cultures all around the world, from the distant reaches, going back many thousands of years. To these cultures, dance was, and is, an invaluable part of life. It's embedded in the human genes, yours included.

In much of the Western world, the scope of dance has become narrow and limited with the theme often being of noisy, unnatural nightclubs and bars. Even music festivals—lined with booths doling out burgers, processed sugar, and alcohol—aren't exactly nurturing, relative to what's possible. But there's a revival of late towards more meaningful dance—dance that takes place in outdoor settings in untainted, natural, beautiful environments, within a real sense of community, much like it was for millennia.

I'd like to share that I'm a part of this new-old tradition. I've become involved in StarTribe (*www.StarTribe.org*), an organization that provides outdoor dance gatherings in northern New Mexico. These events have become quite an attraction. The setting is on a high desert mesa, next to the Rio Grande Gorge and in view of the southern Rocky Mountains. Thousands of people have participated in these events, and for the real spirit of dance. A bonfire built according to ancient Pueblo traditions in the middle of the dance floor creates a magical atmosphere unlike anything else.

The dance and the fire and the music and the setting. There's something very moving and powerful about an entire community of people coming together for this kind of experience. (And you are warmly invited!) Attendees often report feeling a sense of deeper awareness, a clearer view of who they are, a special joy, and a feeling of that awe. I view dance as a martial art of the consciousness, as it has unquestionably helped defend my mind from stress and negativity. A common meditative perspective is that dance is participation with harmony in the Universe. Maybe this is why civilizations all over the world have dance as part of their culture. It's ancient and its benefit is proven. Plus dance is exercise! Ecstatic movement gets the heart rate up for sure. I've made dance a significant part of my life and I can't recommend it highly enough. After all, since we were children, we've been singing the "hokie-pokie" is "what's it all about." Wisdom sometimes has creative ways of making itself known.

Humor

Humor is a medicine. Learn to laugh—especially at yourself. Remember to use your gift of humor in your everyday life. Work to maintain a thread of humor somewhere in your thought. Use it in your dialog with the outside world with the intention to lift up the atmosphere around you. And like everything else you practice, your ability to do so will become stronger.

Pets!

Studies show that people who have pets live longer. They provide a sense of purpose. And even more. When it comes to unconditional love and forgiveness, my golden retriever Arbear has been among my few greatest teachers. And dogs in particular give you one more reason to go for a walk, which for you equals more exercise and sunshine!

Living Environment

Neatness is an important part of maintaining a healthy mind. I've found that un-cluttering my mind and creating a sense of clarity sometimes starts with un-cluttering my home. To a degree, they are intertwined. And I like to add simple things around the house that emphasize positive energy. I have a number of small picture frames visible throughout my living space with little nuggets of wisdom and mini-prayers. The classic, "Be still and listen" is one that I have sitting on my kitchen counter. "Discover your excellence," "You are wonderful," "Gratitude works magic," and "Your life is a treasure," are a few more examples. Get creative and write your own. Little reminders such as these will have great value. And flowers! Studies have proven that flowers can have a physiological influence on the nervous system due to pigments that are unique to a real flower only. These are colors that cannot be fully replicated to have the same effect as the flower itself. We all know the mood enhancing nature of flowers. The fact is, flowers help improve our mental and emotional health. I love contemplating the possible reasons behind it. I suggest always having them in your home.

Stress

Stress is commonly thought of as the boss riding us hard to meet deadlines. But stress is essentially *anything* that puts strain on the mind or body. This includes many things such as lack of sleep, anxiety, poor diet, anger, sadness, and guilt—essentially anything that makes us feel less at ease. The reality is that this is all naturally part of life to a degree.

Stress releases hormones that, short term, aren't such a big deal, as the body knows how to remedy this. But on a regular basis they create as much wear and tear as junk food. And ultimately stress can make the mind and body weaker. Believe it or not, stress is actually proven to be the primary source of all illness. The first thing stress weakens is the immune system, the body's capability of restoring itself. Removing stress so the neurological and immune system can function better is what we're going for.

The idea is how we handle stress, like taking action to remove the common stressful circumstances that come up in daily life. Another vitally important part of reducing the effects of stress is exercise, and more than most people realize. Here's why: stress produces adrenaline. Adrenaline unused leaves the body weaker and the mind irritable and more vulnerable to low moods. So the idea is to "exorcise" the adrenaline, booting it out of the body to leave *everything* stronger at the end, including your natural ability to cope with stress in the future. This is what makes exercise an essential thing for a long life of true well-being. The big picture here is to live a life that reduces the stressors and incorporates restorative anti-stress elements such as a healthy diet, time in the outdoors, *exercise*, esteem-building activities, and spending time with joyous companions.

As we talked about, the mind and the body go hand in hand. A happy body supports a happy mind. Take care of your body so that it can better take care of your mind, and take care of your mind so that it can better take care of your body. You'll be a healthier, happier person. Start thinking of success and prosperity in life in terms of a healthy mind and body. I know we don't like to think of our psychological health being limited by the quality of our lifestyle, but it can be. Do I necessarily think you need to eat healthy to be successful? No. But the mind and body are deeply connected and will empower one another if you make way for it. Besides, soda and fast food weren't around during the days of the ancient mystics and leaders. I'm curious what they would have to say about it, although I have a hunch.

Bottom line: enhanced well-being will be reflected in all facets of your life—energy, longevity, memory, relationships, stress management, general happiness, and more. Let this motivate the full realization of your potential. And what potential is that? Well, when it comes to the power of the mind, the potential is still being uncovered. This is a big question, worthy of contemplation, and imagination too. How about we *really* ponder it together. What's behind our eyes really *is* a universe. And in merely scratching the surface of the inside universe, science can't say exactly what is possible and what the limits might be. Bars are lifted every day as we harness new energy and intelligence that are discovered in us. Let's call it a responsibility, meaning *responding* by fulfilling a way of life relative to what we know will reveal our greatest yet to be. I sense, as you probably do, that collectively, the momentum is building. It's a journey greatly magnified because of the simple reason that we're in this together. Could a new era be born? Could we be on the brink of overriding the notion of impossibility? Let's nurture ourselves (and inspire those around us to do the same) to become great thinkers with ever-strengthening hearts, and use our superhuman (*hero*) powers to see just where we can steer this mighty earth-ship.

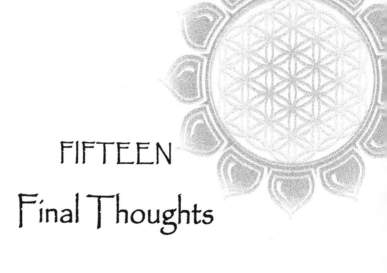

FIFTEEN
Final Thoughts

To Sum it All Up...

I hope, if nothing else, you've come to understand that the material in this book isn't rocket science. I hope you now see that a healthy lifestyle can actually be not so complicated. Some of the material, maybe you already knew. I'm sure on some level you must have been acquainted with the understanding that common diet and lifestyle in the Western world are nuts.

Can you survive on a poor diet with little exercise? We all know people who seem to defy the laws of nature, who maintain a healthy weight yet eat poorly, people who outwardly appear healthy and even energetic, yet pay little attention to what they put into their bodies. Nevertheless, nature always seems to win out in the end, with compromised health down the road. The reality is, there's actually no such thing as cheap food since cheap food now makes the body pay later. And this is about more than just living longer; it's maintaining youth and vigor throughout your life.

I'm confident that your use of the tools we've covered in this book will be reflected in the enhancement of your digestive system, immune system, neurological system, and cardiovascular system—the fundamental pillars of well-being, all of which are linked with everything else in your body. These factors will also be very effective for aiding you in weight-loss, if that's a goal. Now you know the full-spectrum of what constitutes a genuinely healthy way of life. It's really all about having the knowledge and then experiencing the life-enriching value that comes with it.

In this book, we've talked about the right fats and the wrong fats. The processed sugars and the natural ones. We've learned about what defines healthy carbohydrates. The importance of protein and the healthy places to find it. We've learned about the especially important foods like green foods. We've learned about healthy hydration. We've even walked through the course of a typical day's healthy meals. (Hey, if you haven't already, please go detox your pantry! A renewed sense of ease and accomplishment will come with having a clean slate.)

And we've discussed that it doesn't stop there. We've identified how our well-being is affected by sleep, exercise, and sunshine, and how they are synergistic with our diet. And we've defined other vitally important elements that support a strong selfhood. As we've hammered into the ground: all that we do makes us either weaker or stronger. Manifesting the latter with a healthy way of life is not a "sometimes" thing. The influence it can have on your life-force, your very health and longevity, your ability to fend off or heal from disease, and the strength of your mind is nothing less than extraordinary. If you're concerned about the time this takes to gain real results, I would like to remind you that living by the principles herein actually *gives* you time, rather than takes it. Not to mention the quality of life and joy that come with it. Oh, you'll feel it all right!

I said in the Introduction that there's no silver bullet, but, you know, on second thought, actually there is. Diet, exercise, fresh air, sunshine—all of these things *collectively* are what create the silver bullet, also known as life-force. And it's a matter of connecting the dots between this new knowledge and how you live your life. Now that you've read this book, you have an accurate understanding of the way of life that supports a strong selfhood. The fact that you picked it up in the first place indicates you already had the priceless notion about health which puts you in the top percentile.

The limited access to education about healthy living, coupled with the advertising of such things as soda and fast food has given us today's state of affairs, soon to be trumped by wisdom like yours, thus helping remove this burden from humanity. (Our planet will have its sigh of relief too!) Why should we ever do anything again that compromises our body, mind, and spirit? We are not destined to become alienated from our success as a species. Nor will we ever be. I say we rise up in bravery to squelch this feeble paradigm in the name of making way for our greatest selfhood, the potential excellence of which is simply too valuable to waste away in the name of unhealthy entertainment. We are too intelligent to be carried away by ethically poor businesses that attempt to lure us into indulging in health-undermining products and lifestyles. Advertising unhealthy ways of life with healthy looking people is a hilarious irony. Deceitful industry that creates weakness will someday no longer exist. So goes Darwin's theory of evolution.

For the masses it's just been a case of not having the experience of living a truly healthy way of life. Nobody knows what they're missing. They have nothing to compare to their current less-than-healthy lifestyle. Relatively few people know what they can get out of this. But more and more will. And once they live a healthier lifestyle it's hard to go back. It's not only because of feeling better and losing weight. It runs deeper than that. It's because you're tapping into your body's wisdom that is dedicated to unveiling the greatness you were destined to shine. Essentially we are on the path towards coming eye to eye with the *many* wonderful qualities we were born to express. The perspective to maintain here is not so much self improvement. Rather, it's a matter of participation. You're truly ready to just live it. Why not up this journey into hyperdrive? Do it for longevity. Do it to reduce stress. Do it for joy

129

and intelligence. Do it to discover your greatest self and manifest your full potential. Do it to be in your power. The wisdom of how is ancient and in our genes. And it's only a matter of reconnecting with this selfhood, which is what this book has been all about.

Another marvelous aspect of your renewed health is it will be noticed by those around you. Like we talked about in the beginning, life-force is something that others pick up on, and it's very attractive. Naturally you will be a wonderful influence for those around you, making you a light unto a world that needs healing. Experiencing genuine well-being is a birthright. And it's people like you who usher it in. We're all into this together, and having more participation in a healthy way of life will very definitely tip the scales of making the world better too, largely because we will all be better thinkers and problem solvers. And kinder, too. Could we ask for better? This is where outcomes are magnified—things always go better when we work together, especially in the name of well-being.

I believe that within us there is an awesome and very underestimated force wishing to make itself known by the manifestation of something on this planet that is beyond the scope of our current imagination - a similar concept to our present day abilities relative to our abilities just a hundred years ago. Only this time our advance in 'technology', I sense, will involve far more than gadgets. Eighty billion neurons in the brain may just have greater capability than we think. Multiply that by seven billion people on this planet. Now that equates a lot of intelligence. I sense together we are on the brink of unveiling something new that will redefine 'extraordinary'.

Let the life-force we co-generate be the wind in our sails. Life-force has also been been referred to as the human spirit, a symphony of strength and intelligence fueled by the very same source that powers the stars. Excellence is written in our destiny, doorways to which can be found within a healthy mind, body, and spirit. It's love for life and each other that expedites this journey toward claiming our greatest selfhood, and there's no better time to rise to the occasion than now.

Are you in?

Yours very truly, and at your service always,

Billy Merritt

PS. Two more things!...

First, thank you so much for reading my book! Witnessing this content enhance the lives of people like you is what fuels my spirit. Second, if you feel this information serves you, please pass it on to someone you love!

APPENDIX

Recipes for Your New Healthy Lifestyle

Who says eating healthy can't be fun? Not me. And not only can it be fun, it can be delicious and easy, too. Part of my expertise with food is making it both healthy *and* simple. Here are a few of my favorite recipes to get you started. I've organized them by type (breakfast, snacks, soups, etc.), but there are no rules. Maybe you want something under snacks for a meal. (Or vice-versa.) Or maybe you want a smoothie for dessert. Salads can be whole meals and soups work for both lunch or dinner. Try these recipes and eat 'em anytime you like!

What do you say we make the first step here by following through with a detox of that pantry? You know by now the food items you should have in your diet and the food items you should not. Take a close look at what's in your pantry now that you have a better understanding of what constitutes a truly healthy diet. There's bound to be a bunch of stuff you'd be better off tossing. Also since, out of everything in the modern diet, sugar is the very worst (and ironically the hardest to give up) I'd like to make a comment on this one last time. If you have yet to ever completely abstain from sugar for at least two weeks, then *now* is the time. Life is simply too precious to allow something so worthless as sugar to underpin the health of your mind and body. So don't wait! Make the sugar you had earlier be the last. I mentioned it likely won't be easy, but your new knowledge is just what you needed to have the courage and willpower to step up to the plate. I'm confident that you'll be very happy you did this for yourself since the reward you'll get out of it will be anything but subtle.

And remember those packaged flavoring products—sauces, dressings, dips, seasoning mixes. Avoid products with regular salt, and of course, anything artificial or, for that matter, anything that has an unfamiliar name. The question to ask yourself is, are these ingredients from simple, unprocessed foods? Restock your pantry by shopping for products that actually have healthy ingredients by diligently reading those labels. And fats! Chuck the cheap oils that we identified in Chapter 2. Like everything else in your pantry, they are to be replaced with the elites!

Okay. Assuming your pantry is now properly detoxed and restocked, let's get down to the business of preparing those healthy, simple, and delicious meals! Try all of these recipes and then pick the few that you like the most to have on a more regular basis. Remember that we're all a little different physically (we're all unique!) making the nutritive needs of each us at least a little different than anybody else's. Naturally, you'll find that you have your own favorite foods. (Of course we're talking about whole unprocessed foods here!).

Remember the idea that most people of third-world cultures all around the globe often eat nearly the same thing every day, depending on the seasons. Determined largely by climate and culture, their diets are comprised of specific foods that have been in their diets for thousands of years. Naturally, the people of these cultures are physically adapted to the nutritive breakdown of specific foods. Like we talked about, until just a few hundred years ago, eating primarily the same foods every day from the local environment, relevant to the seasons, is the way it was all over the world. And so we all have unique, defined tastes for certain foods deep inside our genes. There will be foods you can select to be a more regular part of your diet that you may never really become tired of, especially when you find tasty ways to prepare them. And there will be foods that you really don't like at all, no matter how they are prepared. This is totally normal and I say trust your taste—it's part of your instincts. Hopefully these recipes will help you think about how to discover what's best for you. Part of the philosophy behind them is that they can be tweaked in any way you wish. Add your own favorite plant foods and spices. Reading these recipes will help you think about how to prepare your own favorites!

SMOOTHIES

▸ *The Ultimate Smoothie – a Perfect Breakfast to start your day!*

BLEND:
1 banana, sliced and frozen (or a pear is a great alternative). If not already frozen then add handful of ice.
1 cup of pure water
1 tablespoon Infinity Greens
2 tablespoons Infinity Protein
2 tablespoons hemp seeds – The key with hemp seeds is to have a high-power blender. Otherwise the better option is 1 round tablespoon raw almond butter.

Amazing! A super-potent alkalizer, body energizer and balanced meal!

▸ *The Afternoon Pick-Me-Up Smoothie*

BLEND:
Half of a frozen pear
5 frozen strawberries
1 cup pure water
1 tablespoon Infinity-C
2 tablespoons Infinity Protein
1 round tablespoon raw almond butter

▸▸ *Banana-Mint Shake Paradise*

ADD TO BLENDER:

1 frozen banana

1 cup pure water

1 tablespoon Infinity Greens

10 drops peppermint extract

2 tablespoons hemp seeds – The key with hemp seeds is to
    have a high-power blender. Otherwise the better option is
    1 heaping tablespoon raw almond butter.

This is total body refreshment!

▸▸ *Coconut Bliss Smoothie*

BLEND IN BLENDER:

Coconut water and meat scooped from fresh Thai coconut.

Simple and amazing.

▸▸ *A Pre-Exercise Smoothie*

BLEND:

1 cup pure water

1 frozen banana

1 tablespoon Infinity Protein

1 rounded tablespoon raw almond butter

This'll get you going!

BREAKFAST

▸ *Classic Oatmeal – a Timeless Favorite*

INTO POT:

1 cup rolled oats

2 cups water

Sprinkle of Celtic sea salt

Cook at low boil for 5 to 10 minutes. Do not stir.

Add 1 tablespoon maple syrup or honey and 1 tablespoon coconut oil or butter.

Add sprinkle of cinnamon

Turn off heat and let stand for 5 minutes.

Stir and then garnish with raw almonds (preferably sprouted) or other raw nuts and seeds of your choice.

This is a perfect breakfast.

SOUPS

▸ *Curried Kale Soup – Simple and Satisfying – and delicious too!*

INGREDIENTS:

2 tomatoes

1 sweet potato

2 carrots

2 cloves garlic

1 lemon

5 kale leaves

1 head broccoli

Indian curry powder

Coconut oil

Celtic sea salt

BLEND IN BLENDER:
tomatoes and 2 cloves garlic

ADD TO POT WITH:
cubed sweet potato
chopped broccoli flowers
5 kale leaves finely chopped (first remove stems)
round tablespoon Indian curry powder
round tablespoon cold-pressed coconut oil
slightly rounded teaspoon Celtic sea salt or salt to taste
Add just enough water to so all chopped ingredients are
   slightly submerged. You can always add more water than
   needed, but the idea is to keep the soup thick and hearty.

Cook at low boil for 20 minutes. Add juice of 1 lemon. Scoop
   1.5 cups of soup into blender and blend until smooth.
   Important: Hold dish towel over top of lid on blender. The
   steam from soup can potentially pop the lid off when you
   hit blend. Also helps to start on low speed.
Add blended soup back to pot and stir.
Add a little water if needed.

▸▸ *Raw Thai Coconut Curry Soup – Delicious!*

BLEND IN BLENDER:
1 Thai coconut (water and all of meat scooped out from
   coconut)
2 leaves collard greens
Juice from half lemon
1 rounded teaspoon Thai curry paste
Sea salt to taste

Yum!

▸ *Raw Gazpacho*

BLEND IN BLENDER:
2 cucumbers peeled and seeds removed
4 Roma tomatoes
1 red bell pepper, seeds removed
½ onion
½ avocado
¼ cup olive oil
¼ cup lemon juice
1 cup carrot juice OR 1 tablespoon honey plus 1 cup water
1 tablespoon dill
1 tablespoon oregano
½ tablespoon chili powder
1 tablespoon dry chives
½ tablespoon sea salt

Add extra water for desired consistency, or a serving of
Infinity Protein for a powerful protein boost.

This is incredibly refreshing on a summer day!

▸ *Spicy Harvest Organic Vegetable Soup*

INGREDIENTS:
2 carrots
½ head cabbage
1 bunch of kale
2 heads broccoli
1 ½ tablespoon chili powder blend
1 sweet potato
½ lb green beans
1 zucchini
3 tablespoons ghee

Chop vegetables into small bite size pieces. As you add
vegetables keep adding water – just enough to cover
vegetables. Simmer until veggies are medium soft.
Scoop approximately ⅓ʳᵈ of vegetables to blender. Add
desired amount of chili powder and blend it up into a
hearty broth. Add back to the pot and simmer to desired
consistency. Salt to taste, if desired.

SALADS

▸ *The Ultimate Salad (and it takes just 5 minutes!)*
This one is my favorite!

Large handful of baby greens into bowl. What is "large" is
up to you. Your instincts rock. Use your fingers to crush/
soften the greens up a little bit. This helps the greens to
better absorb the salad dressing.
Add a handful of sauerkraut
A few sun-cured olives
Five cherry tomatoes
Add a sliced carrot
Quarter cup Infinity Almonds
1 tablespoon ground flaxseed meal
Sprinkle of Celtic sea salt
And why not a dusting of cayenne pepper
For salad dressing – Squeeze one lemon and add 1-2
tablespoons olive oil
Give it a stir and *voila!*
Optional: Add some sliced wild salmon.

Take this one to work. Pack it in a glass Tupperware and off you go!

▸ *Raw Cole-Slaw – Fun to Make and Tasty to Eat!*

For this, you'll need a food processor as well as a blender.

USING SHREDDER BLADE IN FOOD PROCESSOR:
Add 1 head purple and/or green cabbage
2 carrots
1 red onion

BLEND IN THE BLENDER:
½ cup lemon juice
4 tablespoons olive oil
1 tablespoon celery seed
1 teaspoon sea salt
½ teaspoon dry thyme

Mix ingredients together in a large bowl and enjoy!

Here are a couple extra of my favorite salad dressings:

▸ *Tangy Ginger Dressing*

BLEND:
¾ cup olive oil
½ cup lemon juice
2 tablespoons honey
2 tablespoons chopped ginger
1 rounded teaspoon sea salt
How could a dressing be so good? Apply liberally over a
    mix of organic baby greens, sliced avocado and tomato,
    sprouts, and sundried olives.

» *Simply Fabulous Dressing*

BLEND IN BLENDER:
½ cup olive oil
½ cup lemon juice
1 teaspoon sea salt
¼ teaspoon cayenne pepper

Tastes amazing over greens, steamed veggies, or as a dip!

Or, you don't want a salad with dressing?

Then cut to the finish line and just eat a large handful of greens! Like we talked about, greens are vitally important. Who needs salad dressing anyway? Green food doesn't taste bad, so just go for it!

MEALS (LUNCHES AND DINNERS)

» *Red Quinoa with Spinach Salsa Dressing*

PUT INTO POT:
1 cup red quinoa
3 cups water
½ cup shelled edamame
Cook covered at low boil for 15 minutes or until water is
    nearly absorbed. Do not stir
Sprinkle into pot heaping tablespoon chili powder blend,
    teaspoon sea salt and 2 tablespoons of coconut oil. Cook
    for 2-3 more minutes.
Squeeze half of lemon into pot. Give it a stir and turn off
    heat.

ADD TO BLENDER:

½ pound of spinach

¼ cup olive oil

Juice of 3 lemons

Slightly rounded teaspoon Celtic sea salt

2 Roma tomatoes (squeeze some of the juice out first and sauce will be thicker)

½ onion

1 jalapeno pepper with seeds removed (otherwise will be too spicy!)

¼ cup cilantro leaves

Blend until smooth. Serves 3.

This is also a great dip!

Serve quinoa and drizzle desired amount of sauce over top.

Include a serving of baked wild salmon if desired.

This could be your new favorite dish.

▸ *Veggie Wrap – Simplicity and Taste!*
(Makes the perfect quick lunch)

Marinate your favorite leafy greens with olive oil and lemon juice. Or use your new tangy ginger dressing recipe. Sprinkle a little sea salt and cayenne pepper. Roll in sprouted Ezekiel tortilla with sliced avocado and grated carrot.

This is awesome!

▸▸ *Raw Kale Pesto over Quinoa – Easy-Peasy.*

BLEND IN BLENDER:
Full bunch of fresh kale, stems removed
1 tomato
Juice of 3 lemons
⅓ cup olive oil
1 teaspoon sea salt or to taste
Sprinkle of cayenne pepper
Optional: fresh basil

Serve over warm steamed quinoa.

Quinoa for 2: add 1 cup quinoa, 2.5 cups water. Low boil
until water absorbed.

▸▸ *Tamari Rice and Veggies*

½ cup white rice (or brown if you prefer, but white rice has
been in the human diet for thousands of years and is
brilliant) and a little more than one cup water into the pot.
1 sliced carrot
3 sliced Brussels sprouts
2 leaves collard greens, chopped

Low boil until water is absorbed
Broil or boil 6 ounces of cod and add to pot after rice is
cooked
Add 1 tablespoon Tamari and juice of half lemon
3 kalamata olives
1 tablespoon ghee or coconut oil

Stir and serve. I love this one!

➤ *Zucchini Pasta and Marinara Sauce*

You'll need a blender and a food processor for this one.

INGREDIENTS:

zucchini, tomato, sun-dried tomato, onion, bell pepper, garlic, ginger, olive oil, dry basil, oregano, thyme.

Soak 1 cup sun dried tomatoes in 2 cups water for at least a few hours prior to preparation.

To make the spaghetti noodles for 2 servings: use shredder blade and run three zucchinis through the food processor. This will produce noodle-spaghetti-like pieces. Place in metal pot with pure water and add 1 teaspoon sea salt. Heat pot to warm temperature up to 105 degrees (you can just test temp with hand). This will soften the zucchini but allow it to remain raw and enzymatically rich.

For marinara, place the following ingredients in food processor (use blender if you prefer sauce to be smoother):

1 tomato cut in quarters

1 red onion cut in quarters

1 red bell pepper cut into quarters (seeds removed)

1 rounded teaspoon diced fresh ginger

1 cup soaked sun-dried tomatoes

1 cup soak water from sun dried tomatoes

⅔ cup olive oil

2 cloves garlic

1 tablespoon dry basil

1 tablespoon dry oregano

1 tablespoon dry thyme

1 teaspoon sea salt

Strain zucchini pasta and press to squeeze out some of the
extra water. This gives it more of a traditional pasta texture.
Place pasta over bed of greens of choice. Pour sauce over
zucchini pasta and garnish with sun-dried olives and
avocado slices.

Dang this is good!

SNACKS

▸▸ *Zingity-Bling Pesto Dip*

BLEND:
Big handful fresh spinach
1 ripe Roma tomato
Juice of 2 lemons
2 round tablespoons pine nuts
2 tablespoons olive oil
1 teaspoon sea salt
Dash of cayenne

Enjoy with flax seed crackers. Blue corn chips that have
been cooked in coconut oil and seasoned with sea salt are an
acceptable option! These products are out there. Just read
the labels!

▸▸ *Best Guacamole!*

Select avocado of perfect ripeness and scoop into bowl.
Add juice of one lemon and sprinkle of sea salt ... and maybe
a little cayenne!
Mash together with a fork.
Serve with flax seed crackers or celery or cucumber slices.

So easy, so good.

▸▸ *Billy's Green Power Nuggets*

MIX IN A BOWL:
1 cup raw cacao nibs
1 cup hemp seeds
5 tablespoons coconut oil
4 tablespoons raw honey
1 tablespoon Billy's Infinity Greens
20 drops peppermint extract

Mix well and refrigerate for 1 hour
Scoop mixture with spoon and shape into balls (approx 1"
   diameter), and then roll in bowl of hemp seeds. Rub coconut
   oil on hands before shaping nuggets to reduce sticking.
Refrigerate nuggets for at least one more hour.
Serve and enjoy!

BEVERAGES

▸▸ *Ginger Lemon Honey Tea – a Warming Health Tonic*

INTO A BLENDER:
Piece of fresh ginger (the size of your thumb, or you can just
   chop or grate the ginger and stir all the ingredients)
Heaping tablespoon raw honey
Juice of 1 lemon
4 cups water

Blend, strain, heat, serve. Enjoy!

▸▸ *Raw Chocolate Milk*

BLEND IN BLENDER:
Coconut water and meat from fresh Thai coconut
1 Teaspoon cacao powder

Amazing!

MIX INTO 12 OUNCES COLD WATER:
1 round teaspoon Infinity Greens
Juice of 1 lemon
Sprinkle of sea salt
Dash of cayenne pepper
Pure refreshment!

* Why not get creative with your new knowledge and conjure up some new recipes of your very own? Here are four lists of foods to use as a rough guide – those to add, those to have in moderation, those to minimize and those to eliminate.

LIFE-FORCE ENHANCING FOODS

kale
chard
mustard greens
collard greens
spinach
arugula
sprouts
parsley
cabbage
sauerkraut (raw)
Brussels sprouts
broccoli
green beans
peas
blueberries
raspberries
blackberries
strawberries

watermelon
grapes
bananas
pears
apples
oranges
papaya
kiwi
cherries
pomegranate
blue-green algae – spirulina,
    chlorella, Klamath algae
superfoods (research them to
    determine the ones that are fit
    for you)
avocado
sweet potato
carrots

beets

celery

cucumber

squash

pumpkin

onion

lemon

fresh coconut water or meat

tapioca

ginger

turmeric

mushrooms

flax seeds

chia seeds

sesame seeds

almonds

walnuts

pumpkin seeds

white or brown rice

quinoa

oats

beans

lentils

fish we specified in chapter 5

cotton candy (just kidding)

natural spices and herbs, depending. research to identify the best for you

apple cider vinegar

kelp

dulse

and more veggies!

IN MODERATION

millet

amaranth

buckwheat

corn

sprouted wheat

edamame

coconut sugar

chocolate without processed sugar

maple syrup

honey

stevia

mango

pineapple

dried fruit

eggplant

tomato

olive oil

coconut oil

garlic

spicy food

sea salt – Celtic is best

tamari (superior to nama shoyu and regular soy sauce)

cashews

Brazil nuts

macadamia nuts

pistachios

hemp seeds
dairy – yogurt, milk, cheese,
  butter, ghee
goat milk

eggs
tea and coffee – keep it within
  100mg per day

MINIMIZE

pasteurized fruit juice
flour products such as bread, tortillas, bagels, English muffins
products with vinegar
pasta

roasted nuts and seeds
white potatoes
soy products
chicken, lamb, bison, elk, venison, beef & pork

LIFE FORCE DAMPENERS

* *Any* foods containing:
sugar, aka evaporated cane
  juice
high fructose corn syrup
Aspartame
agave
xylitol
iodized salt
hydrogenated vegetable oil
canola oil

peanut oil
palm oil
safflower oil
food coloring
fried foods
anything with ingredients that
  don't sound like food
* Always read the ingredients
  on labels and use your
  wisdom!

About the Author

Billy Merritt has devoted most of his adult life to the study and teaching of natural health and well-being. A frequent guest speaker, he has worked as a mountain-climbing guide and emergency medical technician in Yosemite, and taught nutrition, physical training, and yoga at the world-famous Ashram Health Retreat in the mountains near Malibu, California. But it was only after being diagnosed with a rare and dangerous brain condition that Billy really delved deeply into the connection between lifestyle and health. Today, his condition is in remission, to which Billy credits his diet, his physical fitness, and his lifestyle.

Billy's priority now is sharing his knowledge so that others may learn the simple secrets for living an extraordinary life of health, well-being, and enhanced life-force. He has worked with thousands of people and his research and experience has led him to understand the protocols that he shares in the *Infinity Health Manual*, protocols that go well beyond nutrition and exercise.

Billy lives in Taos, New Mexico, where he operates Billy's Infinity Greens, dedicated to providing elite blends of medicinal herbs and natural superfoods, all of which are known to have significant health benefits, for thousands of people all over the world. Learn more about the Infinity Greens health-enhancing product line and connect with Billy at *www.infinitygreens.com*.